UMBILICAL CORD STEM CELL THERAPY

The Gift of Healing from Healthy Newborns

We are standing at the threshold of a new and exciting medical era, an era of regeneration, rejuvenation, and renewal in which stem cells will set the stage for healing and, in some cases, the restoration of injured, diseased, and debilitated tissues and organs. While stem cell therapy is surely in its infancy, the field is rich with promise.

The debate over the use of embryonic stem cells and the questionable effectiveness of adult stem cells have led many scientists and clinicians to concentrate their energies on umbilical-cord-derived stem cells from healthy newborn babies. While these cells are technically classified as "adult stem cells," they appear to have greater restorative and regenerative potential than stem cells derived from adult tissues due to their young age.

Human umbilical-cord stem cells (hUCSCs) have demonstrated great efficacy in promoting the healing of many conditions. In the last decade or so, pure cord-blood stem cells have been used by physicians to treat a multitude of intractable diseases such as progressive multiple sclerosis, amyotrophic lateral sclerosis, certain degenerative eye disorders, stroke, diabetes, and various forms of heart disease. While certainly no cure-all, umbilical-cord stem cell therapy appears to be amassing a respectable track record in terms of both safety and clinical utility.

In *Umbilical Cord Stem Cell Therapy: The Gift of Healing from Healthy Newborns*, Drs. Steenblock and Payne share some of the science that underlies stem cell therapy and put a human face on this field with accounts of people who have benefited from hUCSC treatments. And, in providing this information, they encourage you to take that bold first step into this vast and wondrous medical frontier.

S0-BZI-130

Umbilical Cord Stem Cell Therapy

Umbilical Cord Stem Cell Therapy

The Gift of Healing from Healthy Newborns

DAVID A. STEENBLOCK, M.S., D.O., AND ANTHONY G. PAYNE, PH.D.

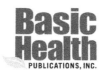

Basic Health PUBLICATIONS, INC.

The information contained in this book is based upon the research and personal and professional experiences of the authors. It is not intended as a substitute for consulting with your physician or other healthcare provider. Any attempt to diagnose and treat an illness should be done under the direction of a healthcare professional.

The publisher does not advocate the use of any particular healthcare protocol but believes the information in this book should be available to the public. The publisher and authors are not responsible for any adverse effects or consequences resulting from the use of the suggestions, preparations, or procedures discussed in this book. Should the reader have any questions concerning the appropriateness of any procedures or preparation mentioned, the authors and the publisher strongly suggest consulting a professional healthcare advisor.

Basic Health Publications, Inc.

Library of Congress Cataloging-in-Publication Data

Steenblock, David.
    Umbilical-cord stem-cell therapy : the gift of healing from healthy newborns /
David Steenblock and Anthony G. Payne.

        p. cm.
    Includes bibliographical references and index.
    ISBN 978-1-59120-125-0 (Hardcover)
    ISBN 978-1-68162-838-7 (Pbk.)

    1. Fetal blood—Transplantation. 2. Hematopoietic stem cells—Transplantation.
3. Cellular therapy. 4. Gene therapy. I. Payne, Anthony G. II. Title.

    RM171.4.S69   2006
    616'.02774—dc22

                                                            2005032200

Editor: Carol Rosenberg
Typesetting/Book design: Gary A. Rosenberg
Cover design: Mike Stromberg

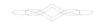

Contents

With love and appreciation to my wife, Noyemy;
daughters, Karen and Amber; and my son, David Jr.
(who is proudly serving his country in the U.S. Army in Iraq),
for their support, encouragement, and sacrifices
in all my endeavors down through the years
including the writing of this book.

I also extend heartfelt thanks to all the researchers,
physicians, therapists, and scores of patients who
have helped transform vision into reality, and theory
into milestones of progress for the betterment
of the human condition.

—DAVID A. STEENBLOCK, M.S., D.O.

Acknowledgments

The authors wish to extend heartfelt thanks to the following people whose direct or indirect input influenced the evolution and content of this book:

Fernando Ramirez, M.D., Director of the Spinal Cord Regeneration Center, Tijuana, Mexico; Paul Sanberg, Ph.D., D.Sc., Distinguished University Professor, Director of the Center of Excellence for Aging and Brain Repair, and Associate VP/Associate Dean for Biotechnology Development at the University of South Florida College of Medicine; Kathy Mitchell, Ph.D., Associate Professor, Department of Pharmacology & Toxicology at the University of Kansas–Laurence; Norman Ende, M.D., of UMD–New Jersey Medical School; Lyn Darnall, M.A., M.Ed., statistician and senior science writer for Steenblock Research Institute; Dave Bloom, President of Bloom Public Relations (www.ournewsroom.com); Sheri Schultz, Ph.D., at Albert Einstein College of Medicine, NYC; Larry Howard, President of Weller Health Institute (www.wellerhealthinstitute.com); and Emer Clarke, Ph.D., at Stem-cell Technologies, Inc. (www.stemcell.com).

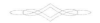

Authors' Note

We are standing at the threshold of a new and exciting medical era—an era of regeneration, rejuvenation, and renewal in which stem cells will set the stage for healing and, in some cases, the restoration of injured, diseased, and debilitated tissues and organs. However, it would be premature to portray this emerging field as "miraculous" or "magical." Stem-cell therapy is surely in its infancy, but it is rich with promise. And though it is buttressed by a tremendous body of scientific work, the therapeutic administration of stem cells is often empiric—meaning that there is often a lot of "give and watch" and "tweak and try again" (more commonly known as "trial and error"). This is a familiar and recurring theme in medicine.

In the pages that follow, we share some of the science that underlies stem-cell therapy and put a human face on this field with accounts of people who have benefited from human umbilical-cord stem-cell treatments. And, in providing this information, we encourage you, the reader, to take that bold first step into this vast and wondrous new medical frontier.

. . . science proceeds as a series of successive approximations.

—EDWIN POWELL HUBBLE
IN *THE NATURE OF SCIENCE AND OTHER LECTURES*, 1954

A Brief History
of Stem-Cell Therapy

The first recorded medical use of stem cells occurred about a century ago when doctors administered stem-cell-rich bone marrow by mouth to patients with anemia or leukemia. Although this attempt to cure or improve these conditions failed, scientists eventually were able to demonstrate that mice with defective bone marrow could be restored to robust health when injected with marrow taken from healthy mice. Quite naturally, this suggested that bone marrow could be transplanted from one human to another.

This process, known as "allogeneic transplantation," was attempted for the first time in people in the late 1950s in France. Patients with leukemia were given doses of radiation that wiped out their marrow, and this was followed by bone-marrow infusions. In many cases, their bodies made new marrow and began producing white and red blood cells, but all of the patients eventually died due to infections or a return of their cancer. All in all, almost 200 allogenic bone-marrow transplants were performed from the late 1950s through the 1960s, but without long-term success. However, transplantation involving identical-twin donors was fairly successful and thus served as a foundation for continued clinical research.

Getting a recipient's body to accept and utilize donated bone marrow was an obvious challenge. In 1958, French scientist Jean Dausset identified the reason for rejection. He found that specialized proteins exist on the surface of the majority of cells in an individual's body, marking the cells and tissues they make up as unique to the individual. These surface markers were dubbed "human leukocyte antigens" (HLA antigens) or "human histocompatibility antigens." It is these markers that make it possible for the immune system to determine what belongs and what doesn't belong in an individual's body. When the immune system encounters foreign markers, or antigens, on a cell, it generates antibodies and other substances to destroy what it perceives as an invader. Disease-causing bacteria, viruses, cancer cells, and foreign matter that breeches the skin are among the "invaders" that the immune system is designed to detect and eradicate.

This surveillance system helps defend the body against things that can cause it harm. This protective mechanism, however, is also behind a recipient's rejection of bone marrow, which carries surface markers that say, "foreign to the body." Therefore, it follows that the antigens on the donated bone marrow must closely match that of the recipient for a bone marrow transplant to take hold. Naturally, bone-marrow transplants between identical twins ensure a 100-percent match between donor and recipient. (Such transplants were among the first to be systematically performed in people.) In the 1960s, as physicians and researchers became more adept at determining HLA compatibility, they began to carry out successful bone-marrow transplants between siblings who were not identical twins.

In 1973, doctors at Memorial Sloan-Kettering Cancer Center in New York City performed the first bone-marrow transplant in which marrow from an unrelated donor was given to a five-year-old child with severe combined immunodeficiency syndrome (SCID)—a rare, usually fatal, genetic disorder in which the body cannot defend itself against germs. The child was given seven successive infusions of marrow, six of which did not fully "take." The seventh finally resulted in engraftment, or acceptance of the donor's cells, and thus brought about the restoration of normal red and white blood-cell-making function.

These early bone-marrow transplants basically brought about improvement in the recipients because of the stem cells contained in the bone marrow. The stem cells went to work in the recipient's bones, creating healthy bone-marrow tissue, which is necessary for the production of red and white blood cells. In the case of leukemia—the overproduction of abnormal white blood cells by the bone marrow—physicians discovered that if the patient's bone marrow is destroyed with chemotherapy (cell-killing drugs) and radiation, they could introduce donated stem-cell-rich marrow that would engraft (take hold) and create healthy bone marrow in the recipient.

Over the past thirty years or so, the use of stem-cell-rich bone marrow, as well as stem-cell-rich umbilical-cord blood, has proven a boon to the treatment of hematopoietic, or blood-related, cancers, especially acute myelogenous leukemia, Hodgkin's disease and other lymphomas, and, most recently, multiple myeloma. This approach has also been used in the treatment of solid tumors such as breast cancer, as well as sickle-cell disease, thalassemia, progressive multiple sclerosis, systemic scleroderma, severe systemic lupus erythematosus, and severe rheumatoid arthritis.

Today, in the United States more than eighty diseases are in some way addressed by bone-marrow transplants and umbilical-cord blood treatments. It is, of course, the stem cells in bone marrow and cord blood that do the work when it comes to actually bringing about the repair, restoration, or healing of an organ or tissue. Logically, it follows that pure stem cells isolated from marrow or cord blood could be employed to bring about more sure or swifter healing responses in ailing people. Bone-marrow stem cells bear HLA antigens that require cross-matching in order to minimize the possibility of an adverse reaction or rejection. Umbilical-cord stem cells, on the other hand, appear to present less of a risk of rejection or adverse reaction. Many studies have shown that even when mismatched cord blood is given to patients, the reaction is generally mild and easily managed. (And interestingly, this immune response to the mismatched blood actually helps patients with leukemia fight their disease.) On the other hand, stem cells extracted from cord blood appear to carry an extremely low risk of rejection or of causing an adverse reaction. In more than 150 patient treatments involving human umbilical-cord stem cells tracked over an almost three year period by Steenblock Research Institute, no such reactions were ever noted. (Growth factors in the vials containing the stem cells did cause some patients problems such as mild muscle tremors, but this side effect vanished once the lab responsible began washing out all the growth factors during the final phase of cell culture processing).

At the present time, the use of cord blood is permitted in the United States for only certain conditions and diseases such as leukemia and anemia (hematopoietic conditions). This reflects a belief among most scientists and physicians that umbilical-cord stem cells are limited to becoming red blood cells and certain immune cells. This commonly held notion is being challenged by a growing body of evidence that cord blood and cord-blood stem cells can help improve many neurologic, eye, and circulatory diseases and disorders, as well, but this proof is tentative and not yet compelling enough to convince the Food and Drug Administration (FDA) to approve or otherwise allow the use of cord blood or cord-blood-derived stem cell for these non-hematopoietic conditions and diseases. Therefore, for the time being, people seeking human umbilical-cord blood stem-cell treatment for neurologic, eye, or circulatory ailments must thus travel abroad to receive this treatment. It is a decisive move that for many is proving well worth the time and expense, as you will soon learn.

CHAPTER 1

Stem Cells:
The Body's Repair Kit

S tem cells—unspecialized cells that give rise to specialized cells—
appear to be one of the body's ablest tools for self-repair. When a
disease or injury strikes, these cells respond to specific chemical signals and set about to facilitate healing by differentiating into the specialized cells required for the body's repair—that is, provided they exist in
sufficient numbers and receive the correct signals when disease or injury
occurs. When they do not, the end result is an inadequate or compromised healing response. With regard to stem-cell therapy, there are a cou-
ple of ways to remedy this: (1) specific tissues can be grown from a
patient's or donor's stem cells outside the body and then transplanted into
the damaged or injured site; and (2) stem cells from a patient or a donor
can be introduced into the body and their activity encouraged by removing impediments to new cell creation and proliferation, such as high levels
of heavy metals, eating foods that support cell growth and multiplication,
and taking select natural or pharmaceutical compounds that support and
sustain these processes. In this way, stem cells can help restore damaged or
diseased organs and tissue. Either way, the donor's stem cells may also
help the body to heal simply by getting it to create certain growth factors
and other body chemicals that promote repair. These remedies are the
essence of true regenerative medicine.

REGENERATION

The realization that certain cells in many, if not most, animals can generate and regenerate tissues and organs is an old one: Aristotle (384–322 B.C.), in his *Generations of Animals* and *History of Animals* observed that salamanders regrow amputated body parts. Around 77 A.D., Roman author and natural philosopher, Pliny the Elder, also wrote about a lizard's ability to regrow its tail. This phenomenon was later mentioned by Dominican friar and famed theologian Albertus Magnus during the thirteenth century. And, in the centuries that followed, many observations were made by various scholars, scientists, and writers concerning the regeneration of limbs by salamanders, of the liver in many animals including humans, of amputated claws of crayfish, and of deer antlers. However, Abraham Trembley (1710–1784) is generally held out by historians of science as having initiated the modern era of research on regeneration. Trembley performed experiments from 1740–1744 involving regeneration in the hydra, a Y-shaped freshwater animal. Some of these experiments included cutting the hydra in half and observing the growth of two complete hydras from the two sections. Trembley found that this regrowth effect also held true when he cut a hydra into four or eight or even more sections. He also painstakingly grafted parts of one hydra onto another and ultimately created a nine-headed hydra, not unlike the Greek mythical creature for which this little animal is named. The "how did it do it?" behind the hydra's ability to regenerate is, of course, stem cells—however, this discovery would not be elucidated until the 1950s with the seminal work of embryologist Leroy Stevens.

Dr. Stevens linked tumors in mice (called *teratomas*) to embryonic cells that lack cell division "shut off" commands that occur naturally in the matrix that houses them in the embryo. Other researchers such as Dr. Gordon Barry Pierce found that once such cells were placed in their native environment (extracellular matric, or ECM), they converted back to normal cells and then went on to become various tissues. Thanks to Dr. Stevens's prolonged, intensive work with teratomas, it was clearly established that they sprang from cells that all others in a developing body *stem from*.

AN INSIDE LOOK AT STEM CELLS

At conception, a zygote (a single cell) is created from the fertilization of an egg, or ovum, by a sperm. This remarkable cell is totipotent, meaning that it is capable of generating every other cell of the human body to make a complete organism. The zygote (the fertilized egg) divides from one cell into two (about twenty hours after insemination), two into four (about forty-eight hours after insemination), and four into eight (about seventy-two hours after insemination). A sixteen- to thirty-two-cell embryo (about ninety-six hours after insemination) is called a morula. This is followed by the blastocyst stage (about one hundred fifteen hours after insemination). Then, cellular reorganization occurs during the gastrulation stage, resulting in two or three tissue (germ) layers as follows: the ectoderm (skin and nervous system), the endoderm (the lining of the gut and internal organs), and the mesoderm (muscles, bones, and heart). All of the cells have identical DNA. However, at this point in development, different genes in different cells begin switching on, leading to the development of the various organs of the body.

Stems cells of the outer ectoderm layer become specialized into brain and spinal-cord nerve cells with their supporting cells called "glia." (The glia help nourish and protect the neurons, or nerve cells, by forming a layer of insulation around them, much like the insulation around electrical wires. The glia form the "white matter" of the brain and the blood-brain barrier.) Stem cells that come from the mesoderm manufacture red blood cells, white blood cells, and platelets, as well as bone, cartilage, fat, muscle, and skin. Stem cells of the endoderm develop into the cells of the digestive system and lungs.

In the early stage embryo, stems cells are pluripotent, which means they have the potential to give rise to every cell and tissue in the body, except the placenta. With the passage of time, stem cells in the various tissues and organs of the body become what scientists refer to as "terminally differentiated," which means they are committed to a specific function. They are thus considered more limited in terms of the kinds of cells they can become and are known technically as "multipotent" stem cells.

Until recently, most scientists believed that differentiated cells could not deviate from their "cellular destiny." For example, it was believed that one could not get an umbilical-cord stem cell to function like a neuron or nerve cell. However, recent laboratory research has cast serious doubts on this contention. In fact, it has been demonstrated that cord blood stem cells can be transformed into cells that behave like neurons. This is of great interest and utility to scientific researchers and the medical community alike.

SOURCES OF THERAPEUTIC STEM CELLS

There are three basic sources of stem cells for therapeutic purposes: embryonic stem cells, adult stem cells (also called "somatic stem cells"), and umbilical-cord-blood-derived stems cells. Let's take a look at each of these.

Embryonic Stem Cells Derived from Aborted Fetuses or Fertilized Eggs

In 1998, it was announced that two teams of scientists working independent of one another had succeeded in isolating embryonic stem cells: One was headed up by Dr. James A. Thomson, an embryologist at the University of Wisconsin, and the other by Dr. John D. Gearhart of the Johns Hopkins University School of Medicine in Baltimore. Dr. Thomson's group went on to develop the world's first human embryonic stem-cell lines. (When a given cell or set of cells is cultured to produce many new generations this chain of related cells is referred to as a "line.") Since that time, much data has been amassed in international clinical studies on these remarkable cells. They have been documented as effective in the treatment of a whole host of medically challenging conditions in animal models, including stroke, diabetes, and certain heart and circulatory ailments. This is due to their capacity to regenerate the blood system, as well as every single organ, tissue, and cellular system.

Although stem cells derived from embryos have shown great promise in terms of their ability to bring about healing or restoration, their use poses numerous technical and scientific challenges, as well as ethical and political ones. (See Appendix A on page 139.)

Adult Stem Cells Derived from Adult Tissue

Adult stem cells, or somatic stem cells, are isolated from the tissues of an adult—for example, from the bone marrow or blood. There are a very small number of stem cells in each tissue, however, so once the adult stem cells are extracted, they need to be grown (cultured) in the laboratory to increase their numbers. The use of adult-derived stem cells is less controversial than the use of embryonic stem cells by far, but it is complicated by the fact that these cells may not afford as much clinical utility as embryonic cells, because they appear to be more restricted in terms of the cell types they can become. And while many adult stem cells can be turned into various cell types in the lab or coaxed to at least mimic other cell types without being exactly like them in all respects, it appears embryonic stem cells have a greater potential to become any cell in the body.

Umbilical-Cord Blood-Derived Stem Cells

Umbilical-cord blood-derived stem cells are harvested from otherwise discarded umbilical cords from natural full-term births. These cells are classified as "adult stem cells"; however, because these stem cells are only nine months old when the cord blood is harvested, they appear to have greater plasticity (the ability to generate differentiated cell types) and thus greater restorative and regenerative potential than stem cells derived from adult tissues.

The debate over using embryonic stem cells and the questionable effectiveness of adult stem cells have led many scientists and clinicians to concentrate their energies on cord-derived stem cells. In both animal and human use, human umbilical-cord stem cells (hUCSCs) have demonstrated great efficacy in promoting the healing of many conditions.

HOW THERAPEUTIC STEM CELLS AUGMENT THE HEALING PROCESS

Many scientists contend that when stem cells are injected or infused into a person, they tend to travel to those parts of the body that have suffered from some type of injury. At these sites of injury, the blood vessels typically have been damaged, narrowed, and constricted. These constrictions prevent the oxygen-carrying red blood cells from passing through to the tissues, which produces areas of reduced oxygen—a state known as "hypoxia." Since stem cells are relatively large, they become lodged in these narrowed and constricted blood vessels (where the low levels of oxygen are just what stem cells tend to thrive in; see "Oxygen and Early Human Development" below). In addition, the endothelial cells that form the inner lining of the damaged blood vessels express certain biochemical signals including cytokines and growth factors, which have been shown in laboratory studies to attract stem cells to the site of damage. Theoretically, once the stem cells arrive at the site of damage, they go about differentiating into the specialized cells required for tissue repair.

Many researchers believe that as the stem cells divide into more specialized cells, they are able to transform into new blood vessels, neurons (nerve cells), muscle tissue, eye tissue, pancreatic tissue, kidney tissue, liver tissue, bone marrow, lung tissue, and so on, depending upon where in the body they wind up and also on the local tissue envi-

Oxygen and Early Human Development

In the early stages of human development, before the first stem cells have become specialized, they develop in a low-oxygen environment. As the embryo grows and the stem cells become specialized, they begin to require more and more oxygen. The more specialized the cell, the greater the oxygen required.

ronment, most likely due to the wealth of growth factors and other body chemicals that influence or govern many aspects of cellular activity contained in the tissues.

CONCLUSION

Ancient peoples observed instances of regeneration in animals, which inspired many ancient myths and esoteric medical practices but also formed the basis of modern research into this field. And, of course, they saw instances of their own bodies' ability to renew and regenerate certain tissues such as skin and bone. Today, we know that at least some of this repair and regeneration is due to the activity of stem cells. Indeed, it appears that these versatile cells are one of the body's most important built-in repair mechanisms. When disease strikes or we sustain an injury or cut, biochemical signals from the diseased, injured, or otherwise traumatized tissue sets the stage for marshalling stem cells to the "hot spot" where they apparently begin churning out compounds that help the body heal and, in some instances, actually are transformed into cells to replace those that are distressed or diseased.

Unfortunately, people's own stem cell supply may not be sufficient to meet the demand posed by a major illness or injury, or else may not respond to signals emanating from the damaged organ or tissue. The aging process may also compromise stem-cell response and subsequent activity, and so may conditions such as heavy metal toxicity that might tend to thwart signal responses or interfere with their ability to migrate, engraft, and proliferate. In these instances, there are medically effective interventions such as heavy metal detoxification and nutritional support that can help make the tissue environment less inhospitable to stem cells, after which stem cells can be introduced into a patient's body to help augment their own native stem-cell defenses. Human umbilical-cord stem cells are prime candidates for this purpose because they have a solid track record in terms of safety and at least preliminary evidence of being effective in helping the body deal with many health challenges.

CHAPTER 2

Umbilical-Cord-Derived Stem Cells

The recognition that there is a connection between blood and healing, and blood and life, goes far back into antiquity. Myths were spun around this, such as the Babylonian tales of blood-lusting vampire-like spirits called Lilitu who prowled by night seeking to find, kill, and drain the blood of newborn babies and pregnant women. This particular myth is compelling because it reveals an early awareness of the life-giving power inherent in blood, especially that of newborns and expectant women. Today, we are fully aware of the tremendous value of blood transfusions in preserving life. We have also discovered that cord blood contains stem cells that can pull off many remarkable medical feats, such as helping to cure leukemia and remedy certain anemias. But how is cord blood collected and given to people with conditions that respond to it? And how do scientists go about removing the stem cells from the blood, expanding their numbers, harvesting, and preserving them? Let's take a look.

THE COLLECTION OF UMBILICAL-CORD BLOOD

The blood from a single umbilical cord amounts to about a thimble or two in volume that contains between 100,000 and 300,000 stem cells. If prearranged with the hospital, the blood is collected from the detached cord within five to fifteen minutes following the birth of a full-term baby. The cord blood is then transported to a cord blood bank where it is tested for communicable diseases such as HIV and hepatitis, processed further, frozen in liquid nitrogen, and stored in a cryogenic vault until needed (see "Umbilical-Cord Stem-Cell Blood Banks" below). The most recent studies suggest that frozen stem cells remain viable for up to eighteen years, if not longer.

THE EXTRACTION OF STEM CELLS FROM UMBILICAL-CORD BLOOD

Stem cells have distinctive biological surface markers (such as CD34 and CD133) that make it possible to extract them from umbilical-cord

Umbilical-Cord Stem-Cell Blood Banks

Once regularly discarded as worthless afterbirth tissue, more and more new parents are opting to send the cord blood or the entire cord from their newborn's birth to a cord blood bank for testing and storage. The reason for this new trend is the increasing evidence that stem-cell-rich cord blood or cord stored today may come to the rescue of a child or family member later in life. This is especially true for families with a history of genetic diseases, such as diabetes or leukemia.

Many experts feel that this "biological insurance" is unwarranted except in cases where families are plagued by certain genetic diseases. However, despite this contrary opinion, in 2005, more than 50,000 new parents signed to have their newborn's cord blood tested and stored at one of the dozen or so private cord blood banks in the United States. In other cases, parents choose to donate the newborn's cord blood to one of the nearly two-dozen not-for-profit cord blood banks in the United States, such as those associated with the American Red Cross or the National Bone Marrow Donor Program. These banks make cord blood available to anyone in need. (See the Resources section.)

blood. These extracted cells are able to (1) divide into two equal cells (symmetrically), thus recreating themselves while preserving their multipotent capacity (self-renewal), and (2) through asymmetrical division, give rise to a variety of functional cells such as blood cells, immune cells, liver cells, and so on that serve a specific function.

New methods of separating umbilical-cord stem cells from blood components that cause rejection (a condition known as "graft versus host disease"; GVHD) have made it relatively easy to produce pure stem cells for use in animals and humans. (See "The Separation of Stem Cells from Cord Blood and Their Processing" on page 17.) The same cannot be said of embryonic and bone-marrow stem cells, or, to

What Do the "CD" and "+"and "–" Mean?

The designation CD stands for "cluster of differentiation," a term that was coined to define cell-surface molecules that were revealed by the action of monoclonal antibodies—that is, antibodies produced in the laboratory that bind to a specific protein or foreign substance. For example, an antibody is created in the lab to a cell-surface molecule such as CD34. When the antibody finds this CD molecule, it latches on. The cell is positive for this CD factor—thus CD34+. When human umbilical-cord stem cells are selected out that are positive for a CD like 34, then we say the resulting collection of cells are CD34+. If cells are deleted that have a particular CD factor, thus leaving behind only cells that lack it—let's say 44—then they are said to be CD44–. Why the numbers, you ask? Clusters of differentiation were assigned numbers such as CD1, CD2, and so on, relating to the order in which they were discovered. In general, each CD is associated with one or more functions, which were discovered through the effects of the antibodies on cell or tissue function.

With input from Steven Goldfinch, Vice President of CureSource, a cord-blood processing and storage firm (www.curesource.net)

a lesser degree, cord blood itself. These do contain elements that can provoke the recipient's body to reject them.

Traditionally, immunosuppressive drugs and radiation have been used prior to bone marrow and cord-blood transplants to lessen the chance of rejection. These pre-treatments are toxic to stem cells and new neurons. Both chemotherapy and radiation are associated with nerve damage and symptoms of memory loss, depression, and declines in IQ. By virtue of the fact that "purified" umbilical-cord blood-derived stem cells (separated from cord-blood components) are safe to use without immunosuppressive therapies, it follows that therapeutic use of these stem cells should be more effective. In short, instead of having large numbers of neurons killed off prior to giving stem cells as is the case with traditional stem cell transplant techniques, patients simply get an infusion or implant of hUCSCs and hopefully build on what they had (neurologically). And this is exactly what's being reported by physicians and researchers involved in treating patients and conducting clinical pilot studies outside the United States.

HOW UMBILICAL-CORD STEM CELLS ARE ADMINISTERED

Umbilical-cord stem cells are generally given by IV, either after a patient's bone marrow has been destroyed (in the case of leukemia and sometimes advanced multiple sclerosis) using chemotherapy or radiation and post-transplant use of immunosuppressive drugs such as cyclosporine to reduce the risk of rejection—or it is given by IV alone.

Traditional Route—Bone Marrow Ablation and Use of Immunosuppressive Drugs

The standard, or traditional, method of performing stem-cell therapy for the purpose of treating blood-related diseases such as leukemia involves destroying the bone marrow of the recipient by use of chemotherapy and radiation, then giving stem-cell-rich marrow or umbilical-cord blood by IV. This approach is risky and requires extreme care to avoid complications, including postoperative infections. (Remember, once the bone marrow is eradicated, the patient's immune system is no longer functional.)

Here in the United States, the National Marrow Donor Program (NMDP) Registry (www.marrow.org/NMDP/registry.html) contains detailed information on more than 5 million volunteer bone-marrow donors and more than 28,000 donated cord-blood units (as of July 2003). The NMDP Registry is the largest collection of such donors in

The Separation of Stem Cells from Cord Blood and Their Processing

One of the most effective ways to remove stem cells from cord blood is with a technique called "immunomagnetic separation." This approach involves attaching ultra-small bits, or nanoparticles, of iron to antibodies that seek out and bind to stem cells that have a particular molecular marker, such as CD34 or CD133. These iron-tagged stem cells and the blood in which they are afloat are then subjected to a magnetic field. The iron-tagged CD34 stem cells adhere to the magnet, while the blood cells and serum and such do not and therefore can be flushed away.

After the blood cells have been drained away, the magnetic field is removed, thereby allowing the stem cells to fall into a waiting collecting dish. So simple, yet so elegant and effective! The stem cells are then cultured in a special solution containing nutrients and growth factors. After reaching a point whereby further expansion cannot be achieved without the cells differentiating—that is, turning into various types of cells—they are harvested, the growth factors are washed out completely, and they are then placed in vials along with a very small amount of a cryopreservative and frozen in liquid nitrogen. (The cryopreservative used is dimethyl sulfoxide [DMSO] and dextran, compounds that prevent the formation of membrane-rupturing ice crystals during freezing.)

the world, and boasts a network of donor centers and transplant centers in fourteen countries with cooperative agreements in existence with fifteen international registries. The NMDP helps coordinate over 170 stem-cell transplants each month and has racked up more than 16,000 total transplants since 1986, when the organization was founded.

Low Adverse-Effects Route: Injection and IV Drip without Radiation or Chemical Ablation of the Bone Marrow and Use of Immunosuppressive Drugs

Umbilical-cord stem cells can be given intravenously (IV drip), by subcutaneous injection, by implant, or by a combination of these approaches. An IV drip takes about thirty minutes, while an injection is completed in a few seconds. Implants including those made into the brain require that patients be hospitalized for anywhere from one day to several weeks. Stem cells introduced by IV drip or subcutaneous injection circulate in the bloodstream where they are exposed to chemical signals such as stromal-derived growth factor-alpha from injured, inflamed, hypoxic (low-oxygen), or diseased tissues. These signals act like homing beacons, calling the stem cells to the area. Implanted stem cells generally are placed into or near the target tissue and thus have little or no migrating to do in order to reach the target organ or tissue.

UMBILICAL-CORD STEM-CELL AUGMENTATION

In order to be clinically effective, stem cells often need to be introduced to the recipient's body in large numbers. Many physicians who perform umbilical-cord stem-cell therapy advocate the use of anywhere from 1 million to 10 million stem cells per treatment. Since a single umbilical cord contains 80 to 220 milliliters of blood and only about 100,000 to 300,000 stem cells, it is necessary to separate the stem cells and then expand their numbers. This is done quite readily in the laboratory by the use of growth factors (substances produced by the body that control the growth, division, and maturation of cells and tissues) and compounds such as retinoic acid (a derivative of vitamin A), making it possible to multiply the 300,000 stem cells in one umbilical cord to more than 10 million cells. This, in turn, can be administered to a patient all at once or in increments, depending on the condition or injury being treated.

Interestingly, a subset of these stem cells bear a unique biological signature, CD133, which has been shown to give rise to white matter, or glial cells, in the laboratory. These stem cells can be separated from other types of stem cells and then used to help the body heal or restore damage or disease in the brain and/or spinal cord. Other subsets that are being utilized clinically abroad include CD44–, which can be coaxed into becoming neurons, including astroctyes and oligodentroctyes, and CD45–, which are deemed "intrinsically pluripotent," meaning they can become many tissue types. (However, researchers do not know yet whether these CD45– hUCSCs will retain this ability once in the human body. Patients have been treated in Mexico with these "intrinsically pluripotent" hUCSCs and their progress is being tracked and analyzed by experts at Steenblock Research Institute.)

Korean scientists recently reported finding that CD34–/45+ could be readily converted into a wide variety of cell types. All these cell subsets are being utilized by the physicians in Mexico mentioned elsewhere in this book to treat neurological diseases and a host of other conditions.

WHAT HAPPENS AFTER A STEM-CELL TREATMENT?

In studies of animals, it has been observed that when stem cells fitted with radioactive tags are introduced into the body and are tracked using radiation-detection devices, the stem cells tend to fan out and show up in various organs, including the brain. This may also be true in humans, as patient responses following stem-cell therapy are consistent with what one would expect to see of stem-cell-facilitated repair or regeneration. Indeed, many people have reported beneficial changes in their conditions during the first few weeks following treatment.

In some cases, improvements after stem-cell therapy begin to

The Safety Record of Umbilical-Cord Blood

Umbilical-cord blood was approved by the FDA for use in certain diseases in the late 1980s. Umbilical-cord blood transfusions, which include a very primitive (and thus biologically versatile) stem cell designated CD34+, have been used in more than 1,000 children and adults since 1986 in the United States. Many of these treatments were administered to cancer patients who subsequently showed significant improvement. Remember, the stem cells in the cord blood are the "active" components used to repair bone marrow and the immune system of patients treated with chemotherapy and radiation. In addition, stem-cell-rich umbilical-cord blood has a seventeen-year track record of being used to treat cancer without causing much in the way of secondary diseases or cancers. It also produces significantly fewer instances of graft versus host disease (GVHD) than bone marrow stem cells and is also easier to obtain.

Cord Blood Stem Cells Deemed Safe

Extract from "Korean Scientists Succeed in Stem Cell Therapy" by Kim Tae-gyu, Staff Reporter, The Korea Times, November 26, 2004

> "Embryonic stem cells are omni-potent in that they can divide into any thing even including a tumor cell. But cord blood stem cells are developed enough not to cause such troubles while retaining as powerful a differentiation capacity at the same time," he [Professor Kang Kyung-Sun] claimed.
>
> Another upside of cord blood stem cells is that they can adapt to the injected bodies without triggering a big negative inner reaction, which are common in other transplantations, according to Han, Ph.D., of the SCB [Dr. Han Hoon of the Seoul Cord Blood Bank].
>
> "We don't need a strict match between cord blood stem cell type and the immune system of a patient because the latter accepts the former pretty well thanks to its immaturity," Han said.

Source: http://times.hankooki.com/lpage/200411/kt2004112617575710440.htm

appear within a day of treatment; however, by and large, it takes two to three weeks to see improvements, with most patients seeing results from the end of the first month through the third month. This corresponds to the period of time it generally takes for the stem cells to bring about healthy changes in the recipient's body through the action of various compounds and growth factors and/or to engraft, or take hold, and bring about beneficial changes in tissues. While some people report experiencing benefits from three to six months or more following stem-cell therapy, most of the improvements appear to plateau and taper off after three to four months.

For those with conditions, such as cerebral palsy, which do not progress by nature, the number of improvements peak at three to four months and fewer gains are seen thereafter. These improvements have not been observed to be eroded or lost, though, because cerebral palsy is not progressive. For people with progressive diseases or conditions like multiple sclerosis or amyotrophic lateral sclerosis (ALS; also called Lou Gehrig's disease), the number and degree of improvements peak at three to four months and few are seen thereafter; however, some (and sometimes all) of these gains are lost or otherwise compromised as the disease progresses.

Stem-Cell Successes

The authors and others at the Steenblock Research Institute in San Clemente, California, have been following the cases of patients treated with hUCSCs, as well as tabulating results from pilot studies performed abroad involving stem-cell therapy for specific conditions such as cerebral palsy in children and stroke in adults. The following are but a few of the many responses documented as of the date of publication. (More detailed case histories are included in Chapter 4.)

- A sixty-five-year-old man with progressive multiple sclerosis was treated with umbilical-cord stem cells in July 2003. Prior to this treatment, he could not swallow water normally. Within a week of receiving hUCSCs, he was able to do so without a problem. He subsequently made noticeable gains in his ability to get around and could communicate more clearly. The condition of his skin also improved. Moreover, as verified by his urologist, a nodule detected on his prostate prior to stem-cell therapy disappeared in the first three months following his treatment. (A more detailed account of this person's experiences can be found on pages 41–44.)

- The Ramirez human umbilical-cord stem-cell therapy program in Mexico has treated more than forty children with cerebral palsy since

Gene-Enhanced hUCSCs for Cancer

In 2005, a line of human umbilical-cord stem cells, into which laboratory scientists inserted two genes, was specifically created for treating cancer. One gene turns the stem cells into tiny factories that churn out interleukin-2, and the other gene, gamma-interferon. (Both of these substances rally the immune system against cancer.) In September 2005, doctors in Mexico began treating terminally ill, end-stage cancer patients with these cells.

Approximately fifteen patients with a variety of cancer types that have spread all through their bodies—for example, breast, melanoma, lung, prostate, and others—have been treated as this book goes to press. Virtually all these people have reported "very significant" reductions in pain and a greatly increased quality of life. Preliminary tests including body scans and biopsies indicate that this approach is bringing about impressive tumor shrinkage and solid tumor die-off. At least some of those treated appear to be headed toward complete remission.

The original idea for this novel approach was made by coauthor Dr. David Steenblock and was subsequently turned into reality by a group of medical school scientists who provide hUCSCs to researchers and research-oriented physicians such as Fernando Ramirez, M.D. (see the Resources section).

March 2003. Eighty-five percent of these children have experienced significant improvements in motor skills and cognitive functions. In one case, a four-year-old boy was cortically blind (a lack of visual functioning despite structurally intact eyes), could not speak well, and could not get around well prior to therapy with hUCSCs. Within seven months of therapy, however, he was able to track objects with his eyes, was beginning to speak, and could move around more ably.

- Jordan Logan, a four-year-old girl, with a terminal genetically based neurological disease called "metachromatic leukodystrophy" (MLD) was treated with 1.5 million hUCSCs. MLD is caused partly by a genetic defect in which a gene critical to the production of an enzyme called "arylsulfatase A" (ARS-A) is missing or not functioning properly. This enzyme makes it possible for a person's body to deal with toxic molecules that we all generate called "sulfatides." Children and adults who do not produce ARS-A or very little experience declines in their neurological function that culminate in disability and death. In children with advanced cases of MLD, improvements in neurological function are never seen and death typically occurs by age five. Prior to the treatment, the girl was cortically blind, her body was limp, and she was on a host of medications. Within two months of her hUCSC injection, however, she could track objects with her eyes and lift her arms and legs high in the air. Eventually, two of the three medications she was on were discontinued.

In late August 2005, the Logan's two-story home in Pass Christian, Mississippi, was flooded and severely damaged by the passage of Hurricane Katrina, a category 4 hurricane. Fortunately, Jordan and her mother, Charlotte, had evacuated to a relative's house in Alabama well before the hurricane hit their community. While all this was going on scientists at a medical school lab had succeeded in inserting a human gene for the ARS-A enzyme into hUCSCs and by doing so had turned them into little factors that produce and excrete the ARS-A enzyme. This approach was first suggested by coauthor Dr. Payne to the medical school researchers who produce hUCSCs that are utilized by Drs. Fernando Ramirez and others in Mexico.

These scientists then went on to create a ARS-A transvected cell line using the highest quality control testing standards followed by careful experimentation involving lab animals. This phase was pretty much complete by late September 2005.

On October 4, 2005, Jordan Logan and her mother were flown to Brownsville, Texas, in a private jet whose use had been donated by a kindhearted, generous businessman named Jim Tatum of Fairhope, Alabama. The following day the Logan's and their pilot made their way to Mexico, where Jordan received 1.5 million of the ARS-A producing hUCSCs. (The cells and clinical services were donated as well.) In the weeks since that historic treatment, Jordan has displayed physical energy and neurological responses not seen since she was an infant. For one thing, she is now turning her head toward people who call out her name. According to Charlotte, this is actually something Jordan has not ever done. She is also now off all medications. And as this book goes to press, tests are to be done shortly that will verify whether the ARS-A enzyme is now showing up in Jordan's blood. Prior tests have shown 0 percent of the enzyme.

Jordan's story has appeared in numerous regional and national newspapers, and has also been the focus of TV coverage in Mississippi. Charlotte is now getting almost daily phone calls from parents of MLD-stricken children residing not only in the United States, but also in many foreign countries such as Canada, England, and Spain. If Jordan Logan continues to improve, virtually all of them plan on going to Mexico to have their ailing children treated with hUCSCs bearing the ARS-A gene.

In a Nutshell: Umbilical-Cord Blood-Derived Stem Cells

• *Since the stem cells are isolated from the umbilical-cord blood, there are no blood cells present, thereby virtually eliminating the need for blood typing or HLA matching. (As you may recall, HLAs are specialized proteins that exist on the surface of cells, marking the cells and tissues they make up as unique to the individual.)*

• *Cord blood-derived stem cells are safer than whole cord blood because there are virtually no instances of graft versus host disease (GVHD) or rejection issues.*

• *There are stem-cell subsets, such as CD45–, that are regarded by researchers as "intrinsically pluripotent," which means they have the potential to become a wide range of cell or tissue types. Whether these cells retain this degree of plasticity in the human body is unknown.*

• *Cord blood-derived stem cells sport a good track record: Cord blood was used therapeutically for the first time in 1988. Since then, a host of laboratory and human-use studies have been carried out that point to the fact that cord-blood therapy is of merit in treating various blood diseases, autoimmune conditions, viral conditions, and neurodegenerative diseases.*

• *In the last decade or so, pure cord-blood stem cells have been utilized by physicians to treat a multitude of intractable diseases such as progressive multiple sclerosis (MS), amyotrophic lateral sclerosis (ALS), macular degeneration, retinitis pigmentosa, stroke, diabetes, and various forms of heart disease. This body of patient responses indicates that umbilical-cord stem-cell therapy does produce clinically significant improvements in many instances.*

• *While certainly no cure-all, umbilical-cord stem-cell therapy appears to be amassing a respectable track record in terms of both safety and clinical utility.*

CHAPTER 3

Improving the Response to Umbilical-Cord Stem-Cell Therapy

As effective as stem-cell therapy seems to be, treatment can be even more effective if certain factors that kill off or compromise the function of stem cells are reduced as much as possible before administration. This includes, but is not limited to, infections or inflammation unrelated to the target organ or tissues one seeks to treat, reducing high levels of toxic heavy metals, and even using some drugs and dietary supplements. In short, the cleaner and healthier the body can be made prior to stem-cell therapy, the better the results are apt to be.

When heavy metals such as lead, mercury, cadmium, beryllium, aluminum, and others are elevated and considered likely to interfere with health, the metal or metals in question must be removed from tissues and the bloodstream using any one or more of various chelating drugs or compounds such as dimercaprol, succimer, penicillamine, desferrioxamine, and edetate calcium disodium (EDTA). Because chelating drugs also can remove beneficial minerals, such as zinc, copper, and iron from the body, doctors typically make sure that these are replaced by use of oral or injected forms of these minerals. (There's more on chelation to come in the section "Reduce High Levels of Heavy Metals" on page 29.)

Infections can often be handled quite effectively with the appropriate antibiotic drug, while inflammation can be quelled using pharmaceutical, natural, and/or dietary measures (depending on the nature and origins of the inflammation, and the degree of severity). For example, the culinary spice turmeric contains a wealth of anti-inflammatory compounds. Analyses of disease patterns in various populations (epidemiological studies) such as the high curry-consuming peoples in countries such as India indicate lower than expected rates of diseases in which inflammation plays a significant role, such as Alzheimer's disease. In addition to eating curry, people can buy standardized commercial extracts that contain the main active ingredient in turmeric, which is called "curcumin." These are sold in health food stores, pharmacies, and grocery stores across the United States.

With these facts in mind, researchers at the Steenblock Research Institute tooled together pre- and post-treatment protocols that have been tested and refined over the course of the past three years (2003–Present). These are being utilized by a number of physicians in Mexico and the United States. So far this approach appears to benefit adults greatly, and especially those with progressive neurological diseases such as progressive multiple sclerosis.

PRE-TREATMENT STEPS

Just as a farmer must till his land, fertilize it, and otherwise prepare it for planting so as to help ensure that the seeds take hold and produce strong, healthy crops, so too must physicians do what they can to make the human body a hospitable place that encourages introduced human umbilical-cord stem cells to find a home, engraft, and begin working optimally. Here is how they go about doing it.

Eradicate Secondary Infections and Inflammation Prior to Therapy

Various studies indicate that stem cells tend to home in on areas of inflammation and low oxygen that typically characterize injured and diseased tissue. It follows that if a person has infections and inflammation in his or her body, stem cells are apt to migrate wherever the "biological fire" is. This kind of diversion can complicate the stem cells' arrival at the target organ or tissue and the subsequent facilitation of the healing process. For example, consider the case of an eighty-three-year-old retired actor who had a stroke a few years before having stem-cell therapy. Just prior to his treatment he began to cough, sneeze, and experience other signs of an infection. He managed to hide his infection from his doctors and went on to receive an infusion of 2 million pure umbilical-cord stem cells. Fearing that disclosing his swiftly developing infection would necessitate antibiotic treatment that might interfere with the stem cells he had been given, he allowed his infection to go untreated. (Sadly he was misinformed; most commonly used antibiotics do not appear to interfere with stem-cell activity or function). Within a short time, he was in the throes of full-fledged pneumonia! However, the pneumonia subsided very quickly, suggesting that the stem cells may have played a role in his recovery, possibly by differentiating into certain immune cells. However, although his lung infection was dispatched unusually quickly, his stroke symptoms remained relatively unchanged. Similar cases have cropped up that underscore the wisdom of eradicating secondary infections and inflammation prior to stem-cell therapy.

Reduce High Levels of Heavy Metals

Doctors in Mexico who perform human umbilical-cord stem-cell therapy typically insist that heavy metals such as lead, cadmium, mercury, and arsenic, which are toxic to proliferating cells, should be reduced as much as possible in the recipient's system. These metals also wreak havoc on the nerve cells in the brain and spinal cord, and interfere with many of the conventional and alternative treatments that patients with neurological diseases undergo.

A physician can run a simple test known as the "DMSA challenge test" to ascertain the level of heavy metals in a person's system. Basically, this test involves ingesting a DMSA-containing capsule. The chemical DMSA binds to certain heavy metals and carries them out in the urine, which is then collected in a special container over a twenty-four-hour period. The urine is analyzed in a laboratory, and the levels of these heavy metals are noted in a report to the physician. High levels are then treated by the physician with the appropriate chelating (metal-removing) drug or chemical.

Eradicate Bacterial Overgrowth in the Gut

Leaky gut syndrome (intestinal permeability) and gut dysbiosis (overgrowth of "bad" bacteria and/or fungi in the gut) should be treated to prevent noxious chemicals called "endotoxins" from entering or otherwise influencing the body and bringing about conditions that might interfere with the activity of introduced stem cells. These conditions are diagnosed using such tests as stool analysis, organic-acid testing, hydrogen breath tests, and gut fermentation profiles. And if a person has a history of intestinal troubles and has consumed raw fish or undercooked beef—or has lived in or visited a country where parasites are often found in meats or fish—then stool testing can be done to disclose whether parasites or their eggs are present.

If gut dysbiosis is present, then the treating doctor will select the appropriate drug, dietary, and/or natural supplements approach for coping with it. If, for example, the cause is an infection of the stomach lining with the ulcer-causing bacterium *Helicobacter pylori,* a course of treatment with an antibiotic such as tetracycline will often be introduced, along with use of bacteria-binding bismuth (Pepto-Bismol) and possibly a natural antipylori agent such as mastic gum. If a patient's intestines have an overgrowth of yeast (*Candida*), then a drug such as Nystatin or Nizoral can be used, along with a diet that restricts sugars that feed fungi, and possibly supplements that specifically kill yeast or compromise their ability to function and churn out toxic compounds (mycotoxins).

When a person has gut dysbiosis, there is often a dramatic increase in the levels of an enzyme called "metalloproteinase 9" (MMP-9), which digests tissue membranes and other structures. This makes the gut "leaky" so that compounds can seep through that are normally kept out of the body. Allergic or immune reactions that can undermine a person's general health can result. The MMP-9 and general inflammation can be reduced using such dietary and supplement compounds as green tea extract, green tea (itself), turmeric root extract, turmeric-rich foods, N-acetyl-L-glutamine, and a host of others.

POST-STEM-CELL TREATMENT CARE

After a stem-cell treatment, there are certain recommendations that should be followed to ensure greatest success. Following through on these recommendations may require the assistance of a physician, therapists, family, friends, or caregivers.

The involvement of a physician is prudent because he or she can keep tabs on a patient's response to human umbilical-cord stem-cell therapy, run tests to access changes in specific organs or in the whole body, and can add, reduce, or eliminate any prescribed drugs a patient is on that might interfere with tissue repair and the production of new cells or tissue.

Reduce or Avoid Stress

It is important that patients reduce emotional and physical stress as much as possible. Stress-induced hormones called "glucocorticoids" produced by the adrenal glands boost the creation of neurotransmitters such as glutamate and aspartate. These compounds are known to damage and even destroy new neurons, and it is conceivable that they might adversely impact introduced stem cells.

Avoid Sugar-Rich Foods

Doctors involved in the hUCSC programs in Mexico and other countries generally recommend that food and beverages high in sugar be avoided. Sugar-rich foods and beverages can cause blood sugar levels to increase and then drop dramatically as the hormone insulin kicks in to counteract this rise. This can trigger a stress response that might have unforeseen negative influences on introduced stem-cell activity.

Avoid Tobacco

Doctors involved in hUCSC therapy abroad recommend that stem-cell recipients avoid using tobacco in any form for at least six months following treatment. Tobacco is sometimes laden with toxic heavy metals and most certainly generates free radicals—noxious compounds that can damage cells. Moreover, the nicotine in tobacco is a poison that can kill cells, including the all-important neurons the nervous system needs to function.

Avoid Alcohol

Because alcohol inhibits the production of nerve growth factor and is toxic to new neurons, most physicians and researchers who perform hUCSC therapy advise patients to avoid drinking alcohol in any form for at least six months following stem-cell treatment.

Avoid Steroids, Opiates, and Grains

The Ramirez Program in Mexico usually advises hUCSC patients to avoid steroids (such as glucosteroids for immune-system suppression) and opiate-containing medications as much as possible and to eliminate grains and cereals from their diets.

Grains, including rice and bread, as well as cow's milk, produce opiate-like compounds called "exorphins" in the body. These compounds appear to play a role in fueling certain inflammatory processes, especially in the central nervous system. If a person has a disease that involves neuroinflammation, such as multiple sclerosis, then eating grains and cereals may exacerbate the problem. (This is akin to throwing gasoline on a raging fire.) More research is needed in this area, but preliminary reports suggest that slower gains are made in patients on predominantly grain diets.

Avoid Allergy-Producing Foods and Foods Rich in Antiproliferative Compounds

Patients who undergo hUCSC therapy are counseled to forgo eating foods rich in chemicals that restrict or inhibit cells from dividing and thus increasing in number (antiproliferative compounds). These foods include many types of berries and citrus fruits such as strawberries, oranges, and limes, as well as fruits such as papaya and pineapple. The consumption of soymilk and soy products and cow's milk is discouraged because these foods are major causes of allergies and also contain compounds that can contribute to the generation of inflammation in various tissues.

Eat Neuroprotectant Foods and Take Neuroprotectant Supplements

People who receive hUCSC therapy are usually advised to eat neuroprotectant foods such as those high in omega-3 fatty acids (like the DHA in fish) and take neuroprotectant supplements such as turmeric extract, folic acid, niacinamide, and N-acetyl-cysteine thirty days or more following their hUCSC treatment. This is because when stem cells are introduced into the human body and begin migrating, engrafting, and presumably multiplying, they need as much protection as they can get to help them survive. The diet focuses on foods high in ORAC value (oxygen radical absorbance capacity). These foods contain high levels of antioxidants known to assist the mitochondria (the cells' energy-producing factories) in pumping out more energy to protect nerve cells from toxic damage and encourage them to thrive and work optimally.

Have a Positive Attitude

Generally speaking, people with a positive attitude seem to improve more quickly after stem-cell treatments than pessimistic people. People who tend to look or focus only on the negative typically need more supervised care to ensure that they do everything in their power to encourage healing.

Patients with mood disorders not requiring medication often benefit from a short course of cognitive therapy. This psychological technique basically teaches people how to recognize and counter negative or overly suspicious thoughts that might run through their heads. Its effectiveness is buttressed by a large number of published clinical studies indicating that cognitive therapy works well in improving mood disorders, paranoia, and anxiety.

CONCLUSION

More than 10,000 babies are born every day across the United States. The cord that sustains them throughout their development contains blood and tissue that is laden with stem cells. Most of these cords are tossed into operating-room waste bins. However, this is slowly changing as more and more doctors, journalists, and laypeople become aware of the "life assurance" aspect of donating or storing cord blood. Science, too, is beginning to move beyond merely collecting donated cord blood for IV transfusions for people who've had their bone marrow wiped out to eliminate leukemia or who need treatment for other bloodborne diseases such as Fanconi's anemia.

Scientists can now readily and easily extract stem cells from cord blood, expand their numbers without use of any animal products or cells (like the mouse feeder cells used to sustain embryonic stem cells in labs), wash away growth factors and such that sustain them while growing and multiplying, and thus wind up with pure stem cells that do not provoke rejection or other adverse reactions in human recipients (no HLA or blood matching is required).

Research-oriented physician Fernando Ramirez in Mexico has been using these "unadulterated" (growth-factor free) hUCSCs to treat various neurologic, eye, and circulatory diseases and disorders for almost three years. With technical input and data collection and analysis from Steenblock Research Institute, certain trends in terms of patient response to these cells have begun to emerge. For one thing, it appears that younger patients tend to reap greater clinical benefits overall when compared to adults who are middle-aged or older. There are also indications that specific pre- and post-treatment measures can help enhance the likelihood that a patient will reduce the presence of toxic heavy metals and dietary factors that interfere with hUCSC engraftment and subsequent activity helps boost patient responses following a hUCSC treatment; as does reducing levels of TIMPs (tissue inhibitors of matrix metalloproteinases), which inhibit a specific hUCSC-generated enzyme called "matrix metalloproteinase-9" (MMP9) that helps these stem cells migrate and then engraft. To this end both pre- and post-hUCSC treatment protocols have been methodically worked out and are being used by Dr. Ramirez's patients, as well as those under the care of many other physicians doing hUCSC therapy in Mexico. The core of this program is embodied in a patent application that was filed with the U.S. Trademark and Patent Office in 2004.

CHAPTER 4

Case Histories

Here in the United States, cord blood is FDA-sanctioned to treat a limited range of bloodborne diseases such as leukemia and Fanconi's anemia, while isolated cord-blood stem cells are restricted primarily to research involving lab animals. This reflects a commonly held notion among U.S. doctors and scientists that cord-blood stem cells can only turn into red blood cells—or in cases in which bone marrow has been destroyed, into marrow that produces red and white blood cells—plus certain immune cells. However, accumulating evidence indicates that umbilical-cord stem cells can turn into a number of different cell types, benefiting neurologic conditions such as cerebral palsy, early to middle-stage multiple sclerosis, early stage amyotrophic lateral sclerosis, and certain eye and blood vessel diseases and conditions. Many laboratory studies, for example, have been published in which hUCSCs have been turned into cells that express specific biomarkers (that is, telltale biological characteristics) common to liver cells, heart cells, neurons, glial cells, and others.

During the course of the past three years, researchers at the Steenblock Research Institute (SRI) have been able to discern certain patterns in terms of how numerous fairly common neurologic, eye, and circulatory diseases treated with hUCSCs respond and to what general degree. Conditions such as cerebral palsy, traumatic brain injury, diabetic retinopathy and neuropathy, and recent stroke have generally shown medically significant improvements following hUCSC therapy, while other conditions have not (see "Responses to hUCSC Therapy by Disease or Condition" on page 94). On the whole, it was found that younger patients tend to show greater positive clinical responses than adults.

What follows is a compendium of patient accounts that includes typical as well as somewhat atypical responses to hUCSC therapy.

MULTIPLE SCLEROSIS (MS)

The brain and spinal cord, which comprise the central nervous system (CNS), are made up of nerve cells. Multiple sclerosis (MS) occurs when the protective, insulating coating around the "wires" that connect nerves (axons) called "myelin" comes under attack. This process leads to a form of degeneration known as "demyelination," as well attendant inflammation in various nearby tissues. In severe demyelination, scar tissue called "plaques" forms along damaged areas of axons. The location, number, and size of plaques determine the type and extent of symptoms experienced. Without proper myelin insulation, electrical impulses from the brain short circuit along the nerve pathway. Axons and nerve cells, or neurons, can also be damaged. CNS-issued commands to the muscles or skin are delayed, confused, or fail completely. In a word, those parts of the CNS that are affected by demyelination pretty much determine the type and intensity of symptoms. For example, some MS patients experience demyelination of the part of the brain that controls thought, sensation, vision, and movement (called the "cerebrum"—the forward and upper portion of the brain). Demyelination here can affect memory, motivation, insight, personality, touch, hearing, vision, and muscle tone.

The cerebellum, lying behind the cerebrum, controls the coordination of movement involving the legs, arms, and hands. The cerebellum also balances the body during walking and running. MS that affects this region can cause sufferers to develop problems in standing and walking.

MS sometimes impairs one or more of the twelve cranial nerves that often causes difficulty in vision, eye movement, speech, swallowing, and, in rare cases, hearing. In other MS patients, the disease process affects the medulla oblongata, or brain stem at the base of the skull, which is crucial to proper eye movement as well as to autonomic, or involuntary, functions, such as breathing, heart contractions, sweating, urination, and defecation.

The spinal cord carries nerve impulses from the brain to the body and a flow of information from the body to the brain. When demyelination occurs in the spinal cord, a disconnection or short circuit occurs that compromises signals to and from the legs, arms, hands, and organs.

The correlation of loss of myelin to signal impairment is not as simple or straightforward as it might seem, however. Symptoms are diverse and vary widely. No two people with nearly identical MS will match up symptomatically. Some people with MS experience severe effects while others report mild ones. Symptoms may be temporary, occurring only during a flare-up or "attack" or they may be continuous. The impact and duration are both unpredictable. This tends to confound both doctors who treat the disease as well as scientists seeking reliable treatments or a cure. Needless to say, this can be very frustrating to MS sufferers and members of their family.

By working closely with a neurologist who stays abreast of new developments and treatments, patients can successfully manage their condition. Many people with MS take medication to reduce the frequency of MS exacerbations, or attacks, and to slow progression of the disease. Prevention of these attacks and comprehensive monitoring and care of the condition are crucial to living with this disease. Most MS patients are able to live fulfilling, productive lives. Seventy-five percent of people with MS never need a wheelchair.

Most scientific investigators believe MS to be an autoimmune disease—one in which the body, through its immune system, launches a defensive attack against its own tissues. So, in MS, it is the nerve-insulating myelin that comes under attack. Some attacks may be linked to an unknown environmental trigger or virus. Still, researchers do not know the exact causes nor have they discovered any sort of cure. And because the symptoms of MS vary and are numerous, scientists and physicians sometimes have trouble even diagnosing this disease with certainty.

Patients with early to middle-stage primary-progressive and secondary-progressive MS treated with hUCSC therapy in Mexico and tracked by researchers at Steenblock Research Institute have shown clinically significant improvements in terms of improved physical and mental energy and the ability to get about, while those with advanced MS typically show little noteworthy responses. How do hUCSCs confer benefit in those who do well? One factor that may be playing a role in facilitating neurologic improvements is "glial derived growth factor" (GDGF). Scientists have found that GDGF nudges myelin-producing cells called Schwann cells to begin producing myelin. Interestingly, hUCSCs express GDGF and may bring about production of other ones such as nerve growth factor. SRI's in-house lab is currently run-

Types of Multiple Sclerosis

The four major categories or types of multiple sclerosis are as follows:

- *Relapsing-remitting (RR) MS—characterized by clearly defined flare-ups, followed by either complete recovery or recovery accompanied by slight loss of function.*

- *Primary-progressive (PP) MS—involves a slow, continuous progression of the disease with only brief episodes of improvement.*

- *Secondary-progressive (SP) MS—starts out as RR MS and eventually becomes PP MS.*

- *Progressive-relapsing (PR) MS—associated with a continuous decline from onset and yet has acute relapses, either with or without recovery to "square one" (the level of MS symptoms prior to the relapse).*

ning tests to determine which growth factors and other compounds are influenced by hUCSC therapy. This should help make explicable at least some of the positive changes seen following hUCSC therapy in both MS and other conditions.

The Jim Haverlock Story

At fifty-three, Jim Haverlock had been healthy and athletic all his life. Illness certainly didn't cross his mind the day he unexpectedly fell while jogging on a South Carolina beach. But when he took another fall a few weeks later, he became concerned. A friend he'd asked to join him on a subsequent run noticed that the toes on Jim's right foot were not flexing properly as he ran. Jim ended up taking another fall that day.

Subsequent falls led him to seek medical assistance, which finally culminated in a neurological diagnosis of a pinched nerve in his back, the probable culprit in his tripping episodes. The neurologist recommended back surgery, but a second neurological opinion in a Charleston hospital negated the first. After experiencing more difficulties with mobility, Jim pursued a neurological recommendation that he seek assistance at the prestigious Mayo clinic.

For ten days, a seemingly endless series of tests were performed at the clinic; Jim was stunned when he was informed that everything had been ruled out except ALS.

After a diagnostic change from ALS to MS, tendered by the late German physician Dr. Hans Nieper, Jim engaged in experimental treatments and personal supplement trials, combined with exercise routines. These treatments included Dr. Nieper's treatment of calcium EAP IV drip, which assists nerve conduction and helps locomotion, and two relatively unsuccessful drug trials that Jim participated in at the University of Washington.

Despite some improvements, over the years Jim's physical limitations increased. Walking was an exhausting experience; he used an electric wheelchair for office and home use, and walked with support canes. His speech, too, worsened steadily, becoming very slurred and extremely labored, to the point that he nearly lost the desire to converse at all; and it became increasingly difficult for him to manage his business and personal affairs.

A merger with friends' businesses allowed him to work part time, when he could. It was a good arrangement at the time, although he was plagued by the need to be self-sufficient and productive. Computers and the Internet were transforming business, making it feasible to earn an income from home. This change benefited Jim further, as he was able to fashion an online venture that began to bring in needed revenue.

Then, in June 2003, through e-mail and phone call exchanges with Dr. Anthony G. Payne at the Steenblock Research Institute, Jim became aware of the medical promise of stem-cell therapy. Jim learned that many progressive MS patients Dr. Payne had been following and working with, who had been treated with umbilical-cord stem cells, were showing clinical improvements, and a few appeared to be headed toward remission.

Jim then spoke further with Dr. David A. Steenblock, the medical director of the Steenblock Research Institute, who very carefully and thoroughly discussed the treatment procedure, consisting of an IV and/or injection done in Mexico, and the expense involved. Jim decided to pursue the treatment and booked an appointment for July 23, 2003, at Dr. Fernando Ramirez's clinic, in Mexico.

Just prior to seeing Dr. Ramirez, Jim underwent a physical examination and a series of special treatments aimed at making the central nervous system tissue environment more hospitable and nurturing for stem-cell graft, while simultaneously amplifying chemical signals emanating from MS lesions (signals that stem cells tend to home in on).

On July 23, Jim met with Dr. Ramirez, who explained the simple infusion procedure. He then thawed the frozen stem cells, drew them up into a syringe, and administered half by IV drip and the rest by subcutaneous injection. The procedure was over fairly quickly, and within a few hours, Jim was back across the border and heading to his daughter's nearby home.

For Jim, the first few days following his treatment brought only a little more fatigue than usual. Then, he found that, although he had previously choked on water whenever he took more than a small sip, he could now swallow in gulps without difficulty.

Prior to stem-cell treatment, his balance had been poor (although it had been somewhat improved by the application of a special hands-on therapy called the Alexander Technique). Thanks to lessons in this technique, he had learned how to coordinate body and mind so he could sit in and rise from chairs without using his arms. After receiving stem-cell therapy, Jim noticed improved balance. With fervent concentration, limited walking without a cane was now possible, and Jim's exercise routine became more doable, improving his quality of life. Because the improvement in his balance following stem-cell therapy required no extra concentration on his part, Jim was convinced that the stem cells were making a difference. But more was to follow!

One of the first symptoms of Jim's MS involved lack of control over his toes. Over time, his toes had curled under from trying desperately to keep a grip on the ground and keep his body upright. They had also basically quit moving, closed in together, and looked very unhealthy.

Shortly after stem-cell therapy, Jim decided to have a pedicure. When he removed his shoes and socks, the pedicurist was amazed to see that Jim's toes had uncurled, straightened out, and were moving independently again, while his skin looked much healthier than it had in the past, so that he could again wear open sandals in summer.

A few weeks after the "toe incident," Jim discovered that he could walk around his home without support, although at a slower pace than "normal." Along with this improved walking ability, friends noted Jim's healthy look and increased energy level. Jim's mood had also improved; he seemed more content, happy, and amenable.

In order to share what was happening with others suffering from MS, Jim added a series of chronicles to a special online MS website he had set up some years before (www.14ushop.com/flyin-blind). His bimonthly entries provide readers with the history of Jim's health, from just prior to stem-cell therapy until the present (2005). The result has been a deluge of e-mails and phone calls. When asked what people appreciate most about his "saga," Jim comments on the hope and encouragement they seem to derive from his accounts.

During the last week of November 2003 Jim contracted and successfully fought off an especially virulent flu virus. His ability to fight off the infection is compelling because people with multiple sclerosis have weakened immune systems, which are more susceptible to being attacked by a wide variety of viruses and bacteria, and are slower to recuperate from them. Jim credits his stronger immune system and his general recovery to stem-cell therapy. (Although Jim's speech worsened after his bout with the flu, it remains improved when compared with his speech prior to the treatment.)

With this litany of improvements in mind, Jim decided that a second stem-cell treatment should give his body some additional "biological mileage." This procedure was performed in January 2004 in Mexico. Following this treatment, his speech and gait improved markedly. There were setbacks wrought by several unfortunate accidents and an infection, but all in all, Jim Haverlock made slow progress in many areas of function. However, his speech did eventually become quite slurred and his ability to walk became so compromised that he took to getting about outdoors in a motorized scooter and indoors with a cane.

In mid-September 2005, Jim once again made his way to Mexico and was given 2.8 million hUCSCs by Dr. Fernando Ramirez. Since that treatment Jim's speech is now much clearer, his sense of balance went from almost "tilt-o-whirl" to very near normal, and he is walking about his home and local malls with less-and-less reliance on his cane. Not surprisingly, Jim has set his sites on doing another treatment in 2006.

The Bill Brachman Story

Bill Brachman, age sixty, is a successful businessman whose world changed dramatically following a diagnosis of multiple sclerosis eight years ago. Like most people with MS, Bill has been through the gamut when it comes to diagnostic workups and treatments; for him, it's a familiar and never-ending story. Bill was even examined by an MS specialist who had dealt with the late Christopher Reeve, and thus was familiar with neurological challenges due to injury as well as to disease.

Bill was told that there was no treatment currently available in the United States that would slow or halt the MS disease process. The best that could be offered were drugs and other treatments that might relieve symptoms and pain and maybe prevent relapses, but none appeared to bring about significant clinical benefits that would endure. For Bill, the best that medicine could offer was disheartening.

One of Bill's greatest concerns was the narrowing in his esophagus, which caused him to choke when he ate or drank. The specter of possibly choking to death haunted him often. Bill also wrestled with slurred speech and episodes of intense shivering, during which his hands would become paralyzed and his speech more slurred. His legs were stiff, and when touched, would shoot straight out and become totally rigid.

In 2002, Bill came across the work of Dr. David Steenblock, president and founder of Brain Therapeutics Medical Clinic and elected president of Steenblock Research Institute. Dr. Steenblock had zeroed in on many of the factors that cause disability and pain in people with MS and had a good track record of successfully managing a great many of these. So Bill forged ahead and had Dr. Steenblock do a battery of tests on him. One of these diagnostic tests revealed that Bill had extraordinarily high levels of mercury in his body—at least ten times the normal level.

Dr. Steenblock explained to Bill that repair is compromised when mercury levels are so greatly elevated. Removing the mercury would require a course of therapy involving chelating (heavy metal–binding) drugs, something Bill readily underwent.

Following chelation and other therapies, Bill touched base with Dr. Anthony G. Payne at Steenblock Research Institute (SRI). SRI was involved in accruing and analyzing data provided by patients, some with multiple sclerosis, who had undergone treatment with pure umbilical-cord stem cells in Mexico; Dr. Payne explained that there was evidence that many of these MS patients had experienced significant clinical benefit after receiving this treatment. This was enough to convince Bill that stem-cell therapy was worth trying.

Following Bill's initial stem-cell treatment in 2003, his difficulty swallowing was resolved, as were the attacks of chills and the paralysis in his hands. In addition, his legs became less rigid. Bill subsequently had two more treatments with pure umbilical-cord stem cells abroad, and reports he has not been able to locate any medication on the market here in the United States that comes close to affording the benefits stem cells have given him.

In November 2004, Bill spent a week at Dr. Steenblock's clinic undergoing special procedures geared to help set the stage for the best possible response to what would be his fourth stem-cell treatment. The regimen Bill underwent included treatment involving various high-tech devices, combined with injection of compounds geared to amplify the signals expressed by diseased tissue. These signals attract stem cells and thus serve as homing beacons.

On November 12, 2004, Bill had his fourth stem-cell treatment in Mexico. Since that time, he has noticed improvements in his speech and less rigidity in his legs. This effect has held fast through the summer of 2005. Bill clings to an informed hope that stem-cell therapy is the ticket to improving his condition and making it manageable and, to this end, was treated again with hUCSCs in Mexico in mid-November 2005. Many people who know Bill feel that the umbilical-cord stem cells coupled with his profound sense of hopeful expectation will work its own magic in his life. It is a familiar story when it comes to interventions on the leading edge of medicine. And it is a familiar story when it comes to the life of Bill Brachman.

CEREBRAL PALSY (CP)

Cerebral palsy (CP) is a neurological condition that affects muscle control. Although permanent, the condition is not progressive. It arises from brain damage or abnormal brain development that primarily affects the nerves and muscles that control body movement and function. This damage or abnormal development can occur during fetal growth, at the time of birth, or within the first two or three years of life.

Anyone who has CP has problems with body movement and posture, although the degree of physical impairment varies. CP can affect the muscles on only one side of the body or on both sides. Uncontrolled reflex movements and muscle tightness, or spasticity, can occur with varying degrees of severity. Some people with CP have only a slight limp or an uncoordinated walk. Others have little or no control over their arms and legs or other parts of their bodies. People with severe forms of cerebral palsy are more likely to have other problems as well, such as seizures or mental retardation. Babies who are born with severe CP may have very limp bodies or, conversely, very stiff bodies. Some birth defects, such as an irregularly shaped spine or small jawbone, sometimes occur along with the condition.

Some babies who are born with CP do not exhibit obvious signs right away. This is why it sometimes seems like CP worsens over time. However, the symptoms simply do not show up until the nervous system matures. Sometimes, a baby may have symptoms that are characteristic of CP without actually having the condition. These symptoms may simply be the result of an immature nervous system and are soon outgrown; or the symptoms may be indicative of another condition. In any event, it may take many months to a few years before a diagnosis of CP can be made.

There is no cure for cerebral palsy. Fortunately, it does not get worse with the passage of time, and the symptoms sometimes moderate with therapy and changes in the body and brain wrought by the aging process and puberty. Standard treatment and care focuses on managing symptoms, sometimes with medications, and maximizing abilities with physical therapy and other special training.

By the early years of this decade, many researchers were beginning to speculate that stem cells might be able to confer benefits on children with cerebral palsy. Animal studies indicated that human cord-blood stem cells injected into rats with freshly induced strokes migrated through the brain's protective barrier and went on to bring about repairs in about 40 percent or so of the affected tissues. "And if this effect held true for stroke," asked many scientists, "might it not also prove true when it comes to cerebral palsy?"

One group of researchers who were asking this very question was found at the Medical College of Georgia. The quest for an answer led

Classification of Cerebral Palsy

Cerebral palsy is classified according to the type of body movement and posture problem involved. These classifications are (1) spastic (pyramidal) cerebral palsy, (2) nonspastic (extrapyramidal) cerebral palsy, and (3) mixed cerebral palsy. Within each of these classifications, there are subcategories.

Spastic (Pyramidal) Cerebral Palsy

CP-related spasticity refers to a tightening of affected muscles without the ability to relax them. Affected joints become stiff and difficult to move. Spasticity is associated with difficulty controlling movements in parts of the body, usually the arms and legs. This can lead to poor coordination and balance, as well as difficulty talking and eating.

There are four types of spastic CP, grouped according to how many limbs are affected.

• *Hemiplegia or diplegia—one arm and one leg on the same side of the body (hemiplegia) or both legs (diplegia or paraplegia) are affected. These are the most common types of spastic cerebral palsy.*

• *Monoplegia—only one arm or leg is affected. Monoplegia is usually a variation of diplegia or hemiplegia.*

• *Quadriplegia—both arms and both legs are affected. Usually the trunk and muscles that control the mouth, tongue, and windpipe are affected as well. This makes eating and talking difficult. Babies with spastic quadriplegia may have problems sucking and swallowing, have a weak or shrill cry, have a very relaxed and floppy body or a very stiff body (when held, they may arch their backs and extend their arms and legs), become irritable and jittery when awake, and sleep a lot or show little interest in what is going on around them.*

• *Triplegia—either both arms and one leg or both legs and one arm. Triplegia may be a variation of quadriplegia.*

Nonspastic (Extrapyramidal) Cerebral Palsy

• *Dyskinetic cerebral palsy is associated with muscle tone that fluctuates between being loose and tight. In some cases, there are involuntary movements of the limbs, face, or torso.*

• *Athetoid (hyperkinetic) CP is characterized by very limp muscles during sleep along with some involuntary jerking (chorea) or writhing (athetosis). If the face and mouth muscles are affected, problems may develop such as unusual facial expressions, drooling, speaking, and choking when sucking, drinking, and eating.*

• *Dystonic cerebral palsy is when the body and neck are held in a stiff position.*

• *Ataxic cerebral palsy is the rarest type of cerebral palsy and involves the entire body. Abnormal body movements affect the trunk, hands, arms, and legs. Ataxic cerebral palsy causes problems with balance, precise movements, coordination, and hand control.*

Mixed Cerebral Palsy

In some cases, symptoms of spastic and nonspastic CP may appear together. For example, spastic legs (symptoms of spastic diplegic cerebral palsy) and problems with facial muscle control (symptoms of dyskinetic cerebral palsy) may both develop.

Total body cerebral palsy affects the entire body to some degree. Complications of cerebral palsy and other medical problems are more likely to develop when the entire body is involved rather than isolated parts. Total body cerebral palsy may include any of the following: spastic quadriplegic cerebral palsy, dyskinetic cerebral palsy, and ataxic cerebral palsy.

these scientists to submit a grant application to the National Institutes of Health (NIH), which resulted in the award of a two-and-one-half-year grant to Dr. James E. Carroll, chief of the Section of Pediatric Neurology (August 2004). Dr. Carroll is employing a mouse model in which an injury to the brain caused by compromised blood flow (ischemia) is treated with bone marrow–derived stem cells placed into the circulatory system.

About the same time Dr. Carroll received his grant, a small pilot study was underway involving eight children with cerebral palsy who had received hUCSCs. This study, spearheaded by Fernando Ramirez, M.D., in Mexico, with technical support from Steenblock Research Institute, involved tracking the response of each child for a period of six months following treatment (with a follow-up six months later).

Each child in the study received approximately 1.5 million hUC-SCs in the form of a subcutaneous injection near their belly buttons, without using drugs to suppress any immune reaction. According to parent reports, none of the children had any adverse reactions whatsoever, such as graft versus host rejection (or vice versa). When the results were tabulated, it was found that all eight children showed some improvement in mobility and/or cognitive function. Six children were rated with improved muscle tone, hip movement, leg movement, rolling to the side, balancing while sitting, and balancing while standing by the end of the six-month follow-up. These responses were underscored by corroborative evaluation reports and statements tendered by pediatricians, pediatric neurologists, physical therapists, teachers, and others involved in the care of many of these children.

One of the most remarkable responses noted during the study involved four-year-old Adam Susser, who was cortically blind due to atrophy of his optic nerves, and who had virtually no chance of ever seeing, according to experts at a major Florida eye institute. Adam began tracking objects during the fourth month following his hUCSC treatment. Adam's parents, Gary and Judy Susser, had him examined by optometrists who found that Adam could indeed see. They proceeded to fit the boy with glasses. He now goes to school and is becoming quite adept at using a computer.

Emily's Story

Emily entered this world in a state of profound oxygen deprivation known in medical parlance as "anoxia," a condition that lasted twenty-eight minutes. As a result of this, she was saddled with profound developmental delays and visual problems and was quickly classified as having cerebral palsy. As she grew older, the extent of her disabilities became painfully evident: She could barely communicate in a way that anyone but her family and therapists could readily understand, she could not count, she was unable to feed herself or walk, and she developed little in the way of a personality. As a result, her five sisters and brothers avoided interacting with her.

In the years that followed, Emily underwent a barrage of therapy in the United States and abroad, which produced modest improvements in her speech and in some aspects of her body movements—though nothing impressive. Among the few seemingly effective treatments were a lengthy series of hyperbaric oxygen treatments (HBOT) and a course of therapy in Poland involving a special rehabilitation apparatus called the "Adeli suit." (This suit is a spin-off of the old Soviet space program; it helps CP patients experience normal posture and movements, patterns that the brain retains as a sort of standard to strive for.)

Emily's parents doggedly investigated and utilized any treatment or regimen that seemed effective. This quest for new avenues led them into the world of stem-cell therapy in 2002. Following lengthy discussions with researchers at Steenblock Research Institute, Emily's parents decided to have her treated with umbilical-cord stem cells abroad. This took place in November 2002.

During the course of the six months that followed, Emily experienced significant improvements in her ability to focus, concentrate, and speak. Her vocabulary expanded dramatically so that she could readily make complex sentences. And her speech patterns improved so much that strangers could understand her. She also developed a greater ability to hold objects such as a crayon than she had prior to stem-cell therapy; and she could also draw a line, count to twenty-four, feed herself, and even make jokes and interact with her siblings.

The kind and degree of positive change in Emily was so striking that her therapists and doctors argued in favor of a second stem-cell treatment. She had this treatment in November 2003, and in the months since that time, Emily has made additional gains in her ability to walk, speak, and interact with her family and others.

Additional stem-cell treatments took place in 2004, and at last report, Emily was getting about using a walker and doing well in her schoolwork.

The Baby S Story

Baby S entered the world healthy, wide awake, and full of vim and vigor. This happy beginning was quickly turned on its head only a few months later when he had a severe stroke that resulted in his being classified by his doctors as having cerebral palsy. The cause? The neurosurgeons, perinatologists, and pediatricians who were called in to determine the "why" behind Baby S's misfortune came up with no answers. Their puzzlement was compounded by the challenge of dealing with a baby who once smiled and reached for toys in his crib, but who was now like a limp rag doll, struggling with medical complications and developmental blocks.

For Baby S, any sound—like a refrigerator door closing or someone sneezing—would cause him to cry inconsolably for twenty minutes or more. The developmental blocks meant that the primitive reflexes that would typically be seen only in newborns would be his lot day in and day out. For example, when startled, Baby S's head would jerk far to the side, and his whole body would stiffen up.

Baby S's primitive reflex problems were complicated by the fact that his head turned to the side automatically and that one arm would shoot out in what is known among experts as "asymmetrical tonic neck response (ATNR) reflex." In a word, Baby S was like a prisoner trapped in a brain-injured body; a prisoner who could not even recognize the presence of the many, festive baby toys that friends and family had set up about his crib.

At six months, Baby S still lacked head control. His fingers were curled tightly around his thumbs, his toes were rigid, and his arms had begun to stiffen up and rotate inward. His legs were basically motionless, and when he cried, his back arched into an upside down "U" shape. Baby S's eyes didn't focus or move well together, and when he was placed on the floor, he would scream out like someone emerging from a very bad dream. His mobility level was estimated to be that of a two- to three-month-old baby—or less.

At one pediatric neurology appointment, Mrs. S. could hear doctors in another room discussing the infant's latest MRI scan results. They were amazed at the amount of damage and exchanged comments such as: "Wow, look at the holes in this kid's brain." Shortly thereafter, Baby S's neurologist came into the exam room and told Mrs. S. there wasn't any hope for her baby to ever be much more than "a vegetable" and that he would require special care for the rest of his life (which might be a short one, given the fact that children this severely disabled are at risk for developing life-threatening complications, such as pneumonia).

Mrs. S. and her husband shared a deep, abiding inner conviction that the neurologist's grave pronouncements were not going to prove prophetic when it came to Baby S, and they promptly sought further medical opinions. A pediatric neurologist on staff at a children's hospital in Utah disagreed with the first diagnosis, stating that the plasticity of the infant's brain might help bring about slow improvements. A pediatric neurosurgeon at a medical school in Oregon agreed.

The Ss focused on seeking out research studies, findings, and even ideas that looked promising for stroke rehabilitation. They also enlisted every therapy service available to them through their state services "Birth to Three Program."

Life became a litany of therapists. The Ss watched as their baby struggled through evaluation after evaluation, typically ending with their being reminded not to expect much for him, save a future of severe seizures and the remote possibility that he might one day be able to interface with the world through technology (computers).

The Ss were determined not to let naysayers have the last word. They fired every therapist who said that Baby S was beyond hope or who treated him like a brainless object that just happened to have arms and legs.

Finally the Ss found a "neurodevelopmentalist" with over thirty-five years of experience and special training in brain injury rehabilitation therapy. This doctor's philosophy—that injured brains could be coaxed into adapting to the injuries and making new connections—made sense. But to do this would take a dedicated team of healers and a lot of determination.

The Ss organized a hand-picked therapy team of doctors and therapists who were highly trained, motivated, and adept at treating brain injury victims. Each team member had to have a specific set of cardinal traits: Hope and open-mindedness. They also had to have experience with helping pediatric stroke patients overcome the odds.

The team of therapists that emerged used their time and expertise artfully to treat Baby S, whom they treated as a person who deserved respect and who they expected would show developmental progress. The immediate therapeutic goal was to maintain Baby's full range of motion, avoid contractures, and give his brain a chance to heal and recircuit as much as it could using integrative treatment approaches.

Baby S's neuromuscular skeletal surgeon worked to address the neuromuscular skeletal issues associated with a body that doesn't move on its own, and proved to be a very open-minded advisor concerning all aspects of Baby's therapy. With her help, the therapy team steered the Ss toward hyperbaric oxygen therapy (HBOT).

HBOT involves placing a person into a chamber where oxygen is pumped in under pressure. Most HBOT center treatments use pressures that are the equivalent to that of about thirty feet below the ocean surface. In the case of babies, mother and child do the treatments together.

HBOT proved a godsend for Baby S: After about fifty treatments (called "dives"), his eyes began to work better, he was able to move his toes a little, and his weak appetite dissipated entirely. Unfortunately, money ran out for more HBOT and the S's fund-raising efforts failed. On the plus side, Baby S never lost any of the progress attained from the course of dives.

After two more intensive years of therapy, including occupational therapy, physical therapy, and speech therapy, the Ss had fulfilled one of their early goals: for Baby S to have a full range of motion without resorting to surgeries, castings, or other prosthetics. This inch-by-inch progress was sufficient to keep the Ss motivated.

Over time, Baby S held his head steadier, and his response to unexpected noises was to cry for only five minutes, rather than twenty-plus minutes, as previously. Clearly, Baby S had overcome the primitive startle reflex and ATNR reflex. And though progress was painstakingly slow, the Ss were seeing the emergence in their son of a happy, sweet personality. He was getting steadily better at recognizing his surrounding environment and was showing an outgoing, playful disposition. Word spread, and in time, many volunteers from the S's church began coming by each day to help the Ss with Baby's prescribed home therapy exercises.

As encouraged as everyone who knew Baby S was by his progress, it was evident that it was happening at a snail's pace. Most alarming was the fact that Baby S's weight had stopped increasing. Because Baby S could not chew, the Ss were faced with the possibility that a GI tube would have to be inserted in order to give their baby enough nourishment to keep him alive.

The Ss wanted to try HBOT again, as they knew of so many children who were having fabulous results with it. While contemplating where to go for HBOT, they heard about David Steenblock. The Ss contacted Dr. Steenblock right away and were told that he would do HBOT on Baby S at a reasonable cost. After successfully checking out Dr. Steenblock's background and credentials with Baby S's surgeon, and consulting the MUMs National Parent-to-Parent Network (www.netnet.net/mums/) and other doctors all across the United States, they learned that Dr. Steenblock was an outstanding physician who was knowledgeable, kind, and on the cutting edge of stroke rehabilitation. Buoyed up by with these glowing recommendations, the Ss made an appointment for Baby S.

While performing an exam on Baby S, Dr. Steenblock shared information and research findings concerning the promise of umbilical-cord blood stem-cell therapy for stroke and other diseases. This rang positive for the Ss, as they had been reading about stem cells and stem-cell research intensely during the year preceding their visit with Dr. Steenblock. As Mrs. S. puts it, "Consulting with doctors at government research centers and other parts of the world via phone and e-mail had become our pastime."

This body of research raised all kinds of questions in the S's minds: Would umbilical-cord stem cells cause cancer like some embryonic stem cells had in lab experiments? Would they do any damage? Dr. Steenblock patiently and carefully laid out the long history of effective use of cord blood to treat leukemia and other disease in adults and children. He also pointed out that treatment with this stem-cell-rich blood had not spawned tumors or other dire illnesses in those treated. And, of course, there were no ethical issues as umbilical-cord stem cells are extracted from placental blood. No embryos or aborted fetuses are involved, which was a major issue for the religious S family.

The research presented by Dr. Steenblock, in concert with that amassed by the Ss on their own, suggested that Baby S might benefit from treatment with pure umbilical-cord stem cells. After considerable prayer and thought, the Ss decided this was Baby S's window of opportunity for improvement. But even if he did not improve, everything they had read and heard indicated Baby S would be no worse for wear for having undergone the treatment. Baby S subsequently received umbilical-cord blood stem cells at Dr. Fernando Ramirez's clinic in Mexico near the U.S.-Mexican border.

During the first few weeks following the treatment, Baby S was exceptionally tired. Fortunately, his neurodevelopmentalist had been briefed on everything and actually had experience with patients who had received stem-cell therapy. The therapist reassured the Ss that all was on track.

Within a month or so following Baby S's treatment, the Ss started to see improvements. According to Mrs. S., "Each day was a little like Christmas because we could see a new improvement, however small, we didn't see before. We saw our baby's progress begin to speed up. In the year following hUCSC treatment, we saw more progress in Baby's rehabilitation than in all the previous years of intensive therapy combined." Among the things the Ss noted: (Note that everything listed below is progress that followed the stem-cell therapy and that this progress has been cumulative. Once a step emerged, it held fast and was "built on" by successive developments.)

August 2003

- Smoothly flexing and extending fingers in succession on occasion.

- Head stability improved.

- Small improvements each week in terms of muscle strength, as well as his ability to employ muscles to do various things (as noted by therapists).

- Able to rotate his wrists.

October 2003

- An increase in joint articulation and muscle tone (without reliance on Botox injections used previously).

- Shows levels of voluntary muscle control in his legs.

January 2004

- Head shape changes (as noted by therapists).

- Invents some simple one-step games.

- Decrease in spasticity.

February 2004

- Can turn his head toward the sources of noise or voices.

- Is engaging in activities that previously would have elicited intense crying.

- Toes and feet are more animated.

- Has started laughing and kicking to propel himself toward toys.

April 2004

- Although still not able to sit up on own, when supine, Baby S can raise his head and upper shoulders a few inches off the floor.

- Shows more upper lip involvement.

- Is much more capable of connecting specific vocalizations to his needs and their satisfaction.

June 2004

- Raises arms occasionally in attempts to reach and grab.

- Brings himself to a sitting position, using arm support, while his legs are straddling an object.

- Brings his hands to midline twice.

July 2004

- Vocalizes something that resembles singing.

- Enjoys greater head control.

August 2004

- Completes a front-back-front roll for the first time.

Oct. 2004
(After second umbilical-cord stem-cell treatment)

- First eats a banana that wasn't mashed up. While holding his hand around the banana (with a little assistance), Baby S brings his head to the banana, takes a bite, chews, and swallows it!

- Rolls from back to tummy and attempts to scoot.

- Enjoys surprises, new sounds, and new people.

- Is a very friendly, curious, and happy, little, wiggly person.

Because the Ss endured years of marginally beneficial therapy, finally seeing major improvements only after Baby S's treatment with stem cells, the S family has come to believe that "the umbilical-cord stem cells are responsible" for the progress.

Mrs. S. adds: "We cannot imagine where we would be without the extraordinary efforts of Dr. David Steenblock, Dr. Anthony G. Payne, and their colleagues at Steenblock Research Institute. We *can* imagine where hUCSC therapy might take our baby. God willing, even though he still has far to go in terms of recovery, the umbilical-cord blood stem cells might ring the alarm clock bell that not only wakes up our baby, but gets him out of bed! All we need is funding for more hUCSC therapy, time, and faith!"

The Alan Robertson Story

When Paul and Linda Robertson first heard the news that they were to be the parents of twins, they were elated. The passage of time quickly disabused Linda of any notion that pregnancy would be fun or exciting: During the pregnancy, she gained sixty pounds and developed gestational diabetes. Then, thirty weeks into it, her water broke and she found herself in an emergency room surrounded by doctors and nurses who were struggling to preserve the health of her babies.

The first baby to make his debut was Alan, followed by Michael. Though small, the boys appeared normal. A little later, the Robertsons were informed that their babies had RDS (respiratory distress syndrome) and had to be on ventilators. Linda, who is a nurse, was well acquainted with what these breathing-aid machines look like and how they work. But nothing prepared her for the sight of her two boys all hooked up by tubes to these mechanical gizmos. Her reaction was immediate: She wept.

Michael rallied quickly; he was discharged and went home after four weeks. But Alan, who had developed an infection, had to remain in the hospital on antibiotics and did not go home for two more weeks.

With help from relatives and time off from their jobs, the Robertsons were able to devote several months to intense one-on-one care of their boys. Soon, although Michael was crawling about the floor on all fours, Alan was having trouble just rolling over. As the months went by, Linda could not help but notice that Alan was not catching up with his brother. In fact, his motor skills, including his ability to get around—were not developing much at all.

The Robertsons promptly took Alan to a pediatric neurologist who did a brain scan. The doctor's findings: Alan had white matter damage to the ventricles in his brain (periventricular leukomalacia), accompanied by bleeding. Diagnosis: Alan had cerebral palsy.

Like other families with special-needs children, the Robertsons' life soon became filled with a litany of therapies and doctors. This was not easy on Linda, especially; she found the whole situation unreal and the source of tremendous grief. Her emotions ran a "roller coaster" course that sorely tested the fabric of her marriage. Paul Robertson, however, held fast and was (as Linda put it), "the anchor that kept our marriage afloat."

Like so many parents in their situation, the Robertsons began researching credible treatments and therapies that might help their son function better. One thing that popped up again and again was hyperbaric oxygen therapy (HBOT). The Robertsons bought a portable home chamber with $12,000 out of their own pocket, and witnessed their son's gradual improvements with regular HBOT at home. They also took Alan to booster camp, a place designed to help children with physical challenges improve their mobility and develop other skills.

Aware of the increasing press and media attention being focused on stem cells, the Robertsons began to more closely examine whether this treatment approach was safe and whether it might benefit their son. While investigating a new HBOT facility in Sacramento, California, early in 2003, Linda learned about some pioneering umbilical-cord stem-cell work going on in Mexico. This led her to www.stemcelltherapies.org and from there to Steenblock Research Institute, where the staff put her in touch with Fernando Ramirez, M.D., and his hUCSC therapy program. After "doing their homework," the Robertsons took Alan to Mexico for treatment in June 2003. In the months that followed, the Robertsons saw rapid improvements in Alan's ability to get about and to manipulate objects. A second stem-cell treatment was done in November 2004. Additional gains in function ensued.

Says an ebullient Linda, "To our great joy Alan has made significant improvements since the two (human umbilical-cord stem-cell) treatments. His muscle spasticity has decreased tremendously, which has benefited his hand dexterity. Before the treatments his hands were usually tightly fisted—now they are open. His right arm was much tighter, but now he can open doorknobs and the refrigerator with his right hand. He can also open candy wrappers, peel off stickers from walls, and do many other things he could not do prior to the umbilical-cord stem-cell treatment. He can now also transition from lying to sitting on his own (something he couldn't do before), his speech has improved, and he usually can communicate in longer sentences than was true before the treatments. And after his second treatment, he was able to walk on a reverse walker by himself!"

The Robertsons' enthusiasm and confidence are palpable; they plan to return to Dr. Ramirez's clinic in the near future for their son's third human umbilical-cord stem-cell treatment.

The Sammy Mograbi Story

Thirteen years ago, Samuel Mograbi suffered a traumatic brain injury at birth from an obstetrical accident known as "abruptio placentae." He was deprived of oxygen for an estimated three to five minutes and was born vaginally (because there was no time to perform a cesarean section), with Apgar scores of 0, 1, and 4. The prognosis was cerebral palsy accompanied by a seizure disorder, and later on, learning disabilities. Throughout Sammy's childhood, the Mograbi family sought and provided Sammy with both traditional and unconventional therapies, treatments, and with education (conductive education)—all with extraordinary results considering the severity of his injury.

Sammy currently attends a private school, accompanied by an educational health aide provided by the school district, and he is mainstreamed in most classes. Sam's aide helps adapt the class work and tests and works with the teachers so that Sam can participate to the best of his abilities. Sammy uses a manual wheelchair in school with some difficulty, and he uses his walker with his aide's assistance. He is verbal with some impairment. Socially, he is age appropriate.

When Sammy was twelve, the Mograbis decided to participate in a pilot stem-cell study in Mexico that was being conducted by Dr.

Ramirez with technical support from Steenblock Research Institute. (Previously, they had had a very positive experience with Dr. Steenblock, when Sammy received hyperbaric oxygen therapy at Dr. Steenblock's Brain Therapeutic Medical Clinic.)

Throughout the one-year period following Sammy's first injection, he experienced some remarkable developmental growth that was documented by standardized evaluations conducted by the Mograbi's occupational and physical therapists.

In Sammy's case, progress has usually been steady, yet slow, because of his CP. Normal development simply cannot and does not occur as it typically does in developing children, but results instead from intensive rehabilitation. Additionally, the progress that Sammy makes is constantly challenged by his physical growth, so that lasting changes are all the more difficult to support and maintain. Therefore, the Mograbis have been proactive in their approach and they support Sammy with a wide range of therapies, treatments, and activities designed to stimulate his rehabilitation. The Mograbis don't feel the need to measure the benefit of each individual therapy as they believe that the variety of therapies presented affords greater opportunities for Sammy's body to integrate what it needs at that particular time.

The first week after the injection, Sammy's mother made sure that Sammy's activities were minimal. Although strict adherence to the required diet was difficult, the Mograbis had explained the cell therapy to Sammy, and he understood the importance of maintaining the diet for at least the first week. Each week, they added a favorite healthy food, staying away from all sweets, beef, and juice for the first month.

After the second week, Sam commented that he felt a little "funny," without being able to articulate what it was: he was aware of something happening in his body. As Sam slipped back into his daily routine, the Mograbis noted subtle, new movements: the way he rotated his left wrist, his right hand now open at rest, the improved dexterity of his left hand, successful attempts to pull off his shirt, and more.

Often, Sammy's therapist had an exciting session to relate. "Shadow" movements were appearing, which meant that new abilities were forthcoming. The cells seemed to be effecting changes at a very low developmental level, at the foundation. Some of Sam's awkward gestures began to smooth out and appear more fluid, as if his awkwardness was compensatory and he revisited earlier stages of development; so that he now had movement options that he did not have previously. The more he chose the correct movement pattern (initially with a therapist's guidance), the more frequent and natural the new movement was. Eventually, he retained the new movements that appeared, and they became the norm. He could now bring his right knee up by himself and maintain a flat right foot when taking a basketball shot, and get himself into the "downward dog" yoga position and do a reciprocal crawl instead of his usual shuffling.

Over time, the Mograbis began to see improvements in Sammy's balance, his fine motor control, and his speech. It seemed as if Sam could better receive and integrate all of his therapies, and there were many; at school, the traditional ones—occupational therapy, physical therapy, and speech—and after school, movement therapy, fitness training, conductive education yoga, swimming, cranial sacral therapy, and massage. During summers, Sam attended the International Clinic of Rehabilitation for a two-week program in the Ukraine, and the Eureca Institute in Anaheim, California, for a four-week Elastic Suit Therapy Program (Grace Wu, owner and director). Sam has worked hard, gotten stronger—and his functional movements have improved accordingly.

As Sammy continued to progress, the Mograbis noticed a change in his attitude; he was more determined than ever to reach his personal goal of independent walking with his walker. In October, one year after his injection, Sammy walked a quarter mile home from his cousins' house. It took him a little over an hour and gave him blisters on his hands, but the look of pride and accomplishment on his face was priceless. The whole family, along with some neighbors and friends, congratulated him! This was a big event in the Mograbi household.

Two months later, the Mograbis returned to the West Coast for a second stem-cell injection. This time the injection was uncomfortable for Sammy and the Mograbis gave him a pain reliever and anti-inflammatory to reduce the pain and swelling at the injection site. After a few days of rest, he felt better and was agreeable about maintaining his diet. Again Sammy told the Mograbis that he was feeling a little different.

Since then, Sam's posture is noticeably straighter, more erect. He says that it is getting easier to do some things because his body is listening and responding better. The Mograbis look forward to seeing what each new day will bring and thank God for the opportunity Sammy has been given by Dr. Ramirez and the other doctors and scientists involved.

The Mograbi family is optimistic about the future. They hope and pray that stem-cell therapy will be the catalyst for healing and improved functional movement for Sammy, and all those with brain injuries, especially the children.

The Tyler and Trent Frye Story

Christy Frye is the mother of nine-year-old twin boys, Tyler and Trent, who have cerebral palsy. The discovery of umbilical-cord stem-cell treatments and the process of obtaining them for the twins has involved the commitment of the entire Frye family—Ron, Christy, and their oldest son Evan, as well as the twins themselves.

The Frye's eldest son, twelve-year-old Evan, is a terrific big brother. At the age of five, he consoled Christy one day by saying: "Don't worry, Mom, if they never walk; I'll just give them piggyback rides!" To this day, whenever feasible, he includes his brothers in his activities. Tyler and Trent, the nine-year-old twin boys who make this story unique, have a super attitude despite having been diagnosed as having spastic quadriplegia cerebral palsy. (A condition that has robbed them of independent functioning.) Trapped inside bodies that will not take them outside when Evan runs by and says, "I'm going to play basketball," they tell Christy that in their dreams, they can run, walk, and play basketball. They will try anything once and never give up despite their disabilities. Christy's ultimate goal is to see the boys walking and functioning independently. If this is never happens, "Evan's back will probably be very sore and tired."

The Frye's journey began in July 2003, when they attended the Third International Symposium for Cerebral Palsy and the Brain-Injured Child. (The boys had previously received eighty hyperbaric treatments, which had lessened spasticity and relieved constipation, thanks to Dr. Paul Harch who would be at this symposium.) At the symposium, the Fryes met Dr. Anthony Payne and learned how umbilical-cord stem-cell therapy being done in Mexico was apparently benefiting children with cerebral palsy and brain injuries. Videos of children before and after treatments revealed significant improvements in motor and cognitive functions. Also at the symposium, the Fryes met Grace Wu, the owner and director of the Eureca Institute, who introduced them to Adeli suit therapy. More aggressive than conventional physical therapy, this therapy involves four to five hours of intensive therapy, using the patented Adeli suit, only available for use by licensed therapists trained in Poland. That spring, the Eureca Institute in California had an opening for the boys, and the Fryes decided to accept it.

During the boys' long therapy sessions at the Eureca Institute, the Fryes remembered the umbilical-cord stem-cell treatments they had learned about at the symposium and, since Dr. Steenblock had an office not far from the Eureca Institute, they arranged to see him. The boys had the heavy-metal testing and allergy tests that Dr. Steenblock suggested; ten well-tolerated hyperbaric treatments were also performed. The Adeli suit therapy proved to be very successful, and the boys were walking on a treadmill for the first time, assisted by the bungee cords.

As the boys' therapy session at the Eureca Institute was ending, with stem-cell treatment very much on her mind, Christy phoned a man (who wishes to remain anonymous) whose wife had tried umbilical-cord stem-cell injections when suffering from advanced multiple sclerosis. During a subsequent conversation, Christy answered his questions about the length of the Frye's marriage, their commitment to the stem-cell therapy and its follow-up, and their religious beliefs. Based on her answers, Christy was elated to learn that he and his wife had decided to donate two injections to the boys! It was the miracle the Fryes had been praying for.

During the next few days, the Fryes discovered that they would be the first of several families to travel to ITL Cancer Clinic in Freeport, Bahamas, for their sons' injections. When they arrived there, Dr. John Clement introduced himself and handed Christy two vials of frozen umbilical-cord stem cells. The moments leading up to the actual injections were difficult for Christy because she was still experiencing the self-doubt that accompanies entering uncharted territory. She had, however, spent more than a year researching different stem-cell treatments and had spoken to other parents who had had umbilical-cord stem cells provided for their children more than once. She wanted what they had—success and improvements. After the injections, the boys experienced slight facial flushing, with Tyler showing some slight redness and swelling at the site of the injection that disappeared within ten minutes. More than physical therapy or Botox, the effects of this type of treatment were immediate and permanent. Tyler's and Trent's spasticity lessened first—they didn't need antispasticity medication or Botox injections anymore. Then about four to six weeks after their injections, to their amazement, Tyler began speaking more clearly—and then, in complete sentences! He still wasn't as quick as his twin, Trent, but there aren't too many kids who can outtalk Trent! Trent's improvements were not as pronounced as Tyler's, since he could already talk and feed himself.

It has been more than a year since Trent's and Tyler's first injection, and the Fryes are hopeful that the results of a second injection might include walking independently. They have just one stumbling block: the need to raise the funds to cover the cost of the stem-cell therapy. Christy hopes that as knowledge and understanding about umbilical stem-cell therapy grows, more resources will become available to treat children with cerebral palsy.

DISEASES OF THE EYES

According to government figures released in 2003, the number of Americans over age forty who will eventually become blind is expected to double within the next two decades. This is due, in part, to the fact that as we age we sometimes develop leaky or clogged blood vessels in or near the retina; we accrue cell damage caused by a lifetime of poor lifestyle choices such as smoking, heavy drinking, and lack of exercise; and we experience tissue damage wrought by the accumulative effects of repeated exposure to strong sunlight and the cell and tissue damaging ultraviolet rays that make it up. As a result, by 2020, almost 6 million Americans will be struggling with visual impairment and loss, according to a special report entitled "Vision Problems in the U.S.," released in 2002 by the National Eye Institute (NEI), a division of the National Institutes of Health.

The risk of going blind or experiencing significantly compromised vision is greatest for people over age seventy-five. The NEI report estimates that half of all cases of blindness can be prevented if the causes are detected and timely treatment is initiated. This should compel anyone over age sixty to get regular eye exams.

According to the report, there are four leading causes of blindness among the elderly:

- Diabetic retinopathy. This condition is a complication of diabetes and basically involves leakage from tiny blood vessels in the eyes. It affects more than 5 million Americans.

- Age-related macular degeneration (AMD). AMD robs more Americans over age sixty of their sight than any other cause. NEI-sponsored research indicates that a combination of antioxidant vitamins and zinc supplements can reduce progression of AMD by 25 percent in people with the most common form of it.

- Cataracts. Approximately 20 million senior citizens in the United States and more than half of those who are age eighty or older have cataracts. Fortunately, this condition is readily treatable with laser surgery and other methods.

- Glaucoma. This is a condition in which pressure builds up in the eye resulting in damage to the optic nerve and visual impairment. It affects about 2.2 million Americans. Glaucoma often goes undetected because the vision loss is noticeable only after significant nerve damage has occurred.

Scores of animal and laboratory studies have been carried out that point to the fact that stem cells can bring about partial or total repair and restoration in many ocular (eye) conditions. For example, during 2003 researchers have successfully transplanted stem cells from the corneal and limbus (the junction of the cornea and the sclera or white part of the eye) into damaged eyes to help restore vision. Using sheets of cultured totipotent stem cells from aborted fetuses transplanted over the eye, scientists have succeeded in facilitating repair with eventual restoration of vision. This technique was used during 2005 (June) to restore the sight of forty patients at Queen Victoria Hospital in Sussex, England, including several with reginitis pigmentosa (RP). One woman with RP who was treated with this transplant had 20:800 vision prior to treatment, and 20:84 two and a half years later. But even so, the success rate of this approach is still fairly low at 20 to 70 percent. Nonetheless, with refinements and additional research, this technique could become a very viable approach to treating blindness caused by disease or damage to the retina, such as macular degeneration.

But embryonic cells may not be the only way to ameliorate various eye conditions. Dr. Ramirez found that simple IV infusions of hUCSCs done at his clinic in Mexico appear to help many people with eye conditions, such as macular degeneration and diabetic retinopathy. Steenblock Research Institute has documented many cases in which very significant improvements followed on the heels of hUCSC treatment. In one especially memorable case, a seventy-four-year-old gentleman who was legally blind in his left eye due to damage wrought by stroke, macular degeneration, and glaucoma, had his vision virtually restored over a six-month period following hUCSCs infused into his body by IV drip and injected subcutaneously around his affected eye.

The Ruth Anne Danbom Story

At forty-six, Ruth Anne Danbom had been a home care and hospice nurse for twenty-five years. Her vision had been affected by fifteen years of diabetes and poor blood sugar control. Since diabetes affects all of the body's systems, the impact was profound. Still, the complications Ruth experienced were relatively rare, especially for someone her age.

Coping with persistent diabetic retinopathy with macular edema, Ruth's healing journey has spanned three years and continues. Her visual decline began as blurring and distortion and rapidly worsened, despite the conventional laser treatment, which at times seemed to make her vision worse.

As recommended by her alternative healing practitioner, Ruth pursued a course of EDTA (IV) chelation to improve the circulation in her eyes and throughout her body. However, very soon after the treatment was begun, Ruth's health was, again, dramatically changed by another complication of diabetes, the collapse of her left foot, a condition called Charcot's foot.

In the local hospital where Ruth sought treatment for her red and distorted foot, she narrowly avoided an unnecessary amputation. No one asked about her vision, which she found had worsened. In addition, Ruth was now prevented from working by order of her doctors.

Ruth's doctor suggested that HBOT might heal the wound created during the exploration of her foot and also improve her vision. She was thus introduced to Dr. Steenblock at the Brain Therapeutics Clinic.

The comprehensive work-up, intervention, and assessments done at this clinic resulted not only in HBOT but also supplementary and dietary guidelines to balance Ruth's whole system. She underwent electromagnetic therapy for her wounds and intravenous chelation with supplements. After five weeks, Ruth's vision improved and she was able to read books for pleasure.

Ruth returned to work, and soon progressed to restricted ambulation with a splint on her now-deformed foot and ankle. About six weeks later, her vision began to deteriorate once more, and Ruth was referred to a new retinal specialist. She reluctantly agreed to the retinal membrane realignment and vitreous exchange procedures he offered her after her insurance company refused to pay the treatments she received at the Brain Therapeutic Clinic, deeming them experimental treatments, not meeting "the standard of care" in her community. The retinologist's overall prognosis was discouraging, and he advised Ruth to apply for Medicare, suggesting that she plan for unemployment and a severely restricted existence.

Meanwhile her position as assistant manager in the Home Health Services and Hospice department was in jeopardy. She was advised by the new department manager that "Unless you can be here one hundred percent, we don't want you to return to work at all."

Ruth then contacted Dr. Steenblock to discuss the options available to her, and he, in turn, referred her to the staff at Steenblock Research Institute for education in what was going on in Mexico in terms of Dr. Ramirez's work with hUCSCs.

To make this treatment possible, Ruth refinanced her house. Then, accompanied by her friend, Ruth traveled first to the Brain Therapeutic Clinic for a series of treatments geared to enhance her response to hUCSC therapy. Treatments there were twice a day for the three days prior to the administration of the cells. While there, Dr. Steenblock advised Ruth that the white spots that had appeared on her left, small toe might be an infection; Ruth planned to follow up with her podiatrist, on returning home.

Ruth was then driven to the clinic in Mexico where Dr. Ramirez fully explained the treatment and his credentials and cited results of the stem-cell treatments, which she found impressive. Then, the cord-blood stem cells were injected on the side of her face and eyes in two injections. She received growth factors subcutaneously in her abdomen. The long-awaited procedure was completed in about a half hour.

Ruth protected her eyes and head from direct sun on the trip home, as instructed. Back home, her podiatrist told her that the white spots noted at the clinic were fractured toe bones, caused by a bone infection, osteomyelitis. Amputation was again a possibility if antibiotics did not help resolve the infection. After the podiatrist checked with Dr. Steenblock about the choice of antibiotics, Ruth began what would be six months of dual-agent antibiotic therapy.

Sometime early in the summer Ruth realized that she no longer suffered from irritable bowel syndrome—an unintended healing possibly resulting from the stem-cell treatment. Meanwhile, subsequent visits to her podiatrist included x-rays to monitor the osteomyelitis. The infection dissolved the far end of one bone, but the remaining jagged portion of the fracture area rounded over and did not require mechanical smoothing by surgery.

More exciting was the change in the structure of the metatarsal bones. After the Charcot's foot acute collapse, these bones had showed up on x-ray like a fading rainbow of osteoporosis with the fifth metatarsal being the most ghostlike. Now, since the stem cells, the bones all appeared to have full structural integrity. The bone infection healed and amputation was averted.

At the end of the summer, the retinologist at last released Ruth to return to work. Although an evaluator deemed that testing using adaptive equipment indicated that Ruth could return to her desk job, the hospital declined to return Ruth to her usual position. Ruth agreed to a part-time position working alone on the weekends as the intake co-coordinator in order to retain her health insurance.

Ruth found it was helpful to use the magnification systems on a routine basis for the first month or two. After that, she began to be able to read even small type without that assistance. Ruth has not achieved 20/20 vision to date. Because of the two areas of acute inflammation (bowel and toe), it is supposed that the stem cells migrated predominately to those areas despite where they had been administered. Ruth concludes that continence and avoidance of amputation are worthy and valuable results of the cord-blood stem cells she received.

Now, two years after receiving stem cells, the spots in Ruth's vision have disappeared, and she experiences fewer visual distortions. Most recently, she has been able to read her writing and view the computer screen without removing her long-distance glasses.

Ruth speaks out regularly on the popular desire for medicine and cutting-edge science to be more in step and more responsive to our hopes for improvement in our daily lives. Both fields move slowly; for those with chronic health challenges, the waiting seems wasteful when there are so many promising findings being reported.

The Katya Dvorak Story

When their daughter was born thirteen years ago, the Dvoraks suddenly became one of those families no one wants to be. They enjoyed two days of bliss as Katya seemingly slept peacefully—their concerns that she wasn't interested in eating were waved away by the nurses and other professionals as normal. They took her home, and it was only when her mother, Cheryl, was left alone with Katya that she could see there was something very wrong. They rushed Katya back to the hospital—and stepped into twelve years of a neurological, dysfunctional nightmare.

There was brain damage, but because medical science still knew relatively little about the brain (according to the director of the neurology department), the physicians couldn't pinpoint it and didn't know the cause or the extent of the damage. The Dvoraks were pretty much on their own in a world of doctors shrugging their shoulders and saying things like "only about 10 percent of babies like your daughter grow developmentally beyond where she is right now." Cheryl walked out the door and never looked back. If there was a 10 percent chance, Katya would be in that 10 percent; if medicine could offer the Dvoraks only dire predictions because it had no answers, they would seek out avenues where hope resided. Day after day in the Newborn Intensive Care Unit (NBICU) Cheryl prayed for her daughter to live and vowed she would do whatever was needed to help Katya find her life. Katya did live through those early months, and they took her home.

Twelve years of struggle went by. Trying all the available therapies that work "from the outside in" wiped the Dvoraks out financially and emotionally and didn't seem to inspire any real motivation in Katya. Katya couldn't do anything for herself physically, and Cheryl could find little, if any, will in her daughter to move forward. Cheryl seemed to be guiding everything: her hope for Katya to speak and walk, her vision for her daughter to have an independent life. Cheryl even started a

72

school for her based on the best "therapy" she had discovered over twelve years of research, but Katya just seemed to go through the motions, and everything—even merely holding her head upright—was an immense struggle for her. Cheryl wondered if she was hopelessly forcing her daughter to go through these exercises; she felt there was a person inside Katya who wanted to grow but who didn't have the means to do so.

Cheryl had heard of stem cells when Katya was an infant, and it wasn't a giant leap to conclude that with stem cells Katya's brain might heal and she might make the most dramatic growth possible: Of course "from the inside out" was the best answer! Cheryl annually checked with a doctor at Stanford University to ask about stem-cell trials Katya might participate in, and was told to check back in two years. The biggest heartbreak lay in knowing that this path was the only hope that Katya might someday guide her own life, and it was out of the family's reach. Why couldn't stem-cell research be put at the forefront of all medical research? It was obvious to Cheryl that it would help millions of suffering people and families!

The summer of 2003 was very hard. The Dvoraks were worn out; Katya was sick more often than usual and wasn't able to do anything the Dvoraks asked of her at their school. It had been twelve years and the Dvorak's daughter still couldn't walk, talk, or communicate yes or no, hold anything in her hand, sit, stand, roll over, feed herself, or eat food (she was administered liquids through a gastrostomy-tube or G-tube) plugged into her stomach. She seemed to be losing any ground she had gained.

Then someone handed Cheryl a website about stem-cell biology and published research. It concerned Dr. Ramirez's ongoing work in Mexico. It was fairly expensive and the Dvoraks had no idea how they were going to make it happen, but Cheryl knew they had to—this was what she had waited for all of Katya's life. She prayed for the price to come down. Miraculously, a few weeks later she received an invitation for Katya to be a part of a pilot study going on in Mexico in which eight children were ultimately to be admitted and charged a nominal fee.

Cheryl weeps as she relates the day that Katya received her first stem-cell infusion—December 4, 2003, which now seems like Katya's true birth date. The progress the Dvoraks had been seeking for twelve years immediately began to emerge. One week after the procedure, the Dvoraks noticed significant changes in Katya. Her thought processes firing up seemed almost visible; she was acting more aware as if processing her environment more keenly, and she would occasionally have little epiphanies, as if something had suddenly grabbed her attention; then she would react by looking thrilled and happy and giggling. Katya was more attentive to the Dvoraks as well, and was making better eye contact.

Physically, Katya began to use her body differently and more effectively. Her movements and positioning of her body were less rigid. Before stem cells, Katya rotated her left leg inward so rigidly it was hard to move it at all. She would often torque her back into a stiff arch, and she always held her shoulders and arms very tightly, without any fluidity. Right after the first treatment, her body became softer, and the Dvoraks had initial concerns that she might lose the movements she had learned, because kids with cerebral palsy learn to move inappropriately from birth, by tensing their bodies into contorted patterns in order to get from point A to point B. For example, in doing a transfer from her wheelchair to her toilet, bed or floor, Katya had learned over the years to abruptly thrust herself upright, throwing her back and head into a backward arch. Now, her body became soft, as if she wasn't sure what to do to stand up. The Dvoraks thought that these less rigid, explosive, and apparently more deliberate movements meant that Kayta was using her body more effectively. The arch in her lower back was less pronounced, and her left leg could be moved more easily and in more coordinated ways during therapy. (One year later, this has corrected itself and she is again helping with transfers by standing up, now with more anticipation and balance, less rigidity, and more thought behind her actions.)

Katya still exhibits rigidity when working at tasks—she tries too hard to do things, but again her thinking seems visible as she makes the attempt. Also immediately after the first treatment, Katya's therapist reported more balanced sitting, and Katya was assisting therapy on the therapist's request with less delay time. So Katya began processing information faster right from the beginning of stem-cell infusion. And everyone noticed that she now used her arms and hands with more purpose. She reached out and grabbed more deliberately, and this was accompanied by more concentrated eye contact with objects.

The growing articulation of body movements developed slowly and steadily throughout the six months after her first stem-cell infusion. This development was accompanied by a more overall conscious presence and more attempts at communication than the Dvoraks had seen in twelve years!

After three months, Katya's overall tone continued to be more relaxed and less compensatory. Her ability to do requested tasks and movements, such as balanced sitting, and maintaining a sitting position, improved. Before stem-cell therapy, her jerky movements would unbalance her and outside noises would make her jump. Now she was more present and attempted more conscious, meaningful responses when spoken to. Her understanding and memory seemed greater. She developed more skills in the use of her arms and hands: she no longer required liquid supplementation through her feeding tube and was finally able to consume solid food orally. She held her own spoon and brought it to her mouth.

Katya still could not regain her balance when it was thrown off, nor could she talk, but she had increased vocalizations and intonations in ways that seemed meaningful to her, and added more varied sounds to her "vocabulary."

After six months, Katya not only held onto her spoon, but could dip it into her bowl, making sure the spoon scraped the bowl, and then lift it to her mouth. Then and now (six months later), it is only due to time constraints that Cheryl continues to put the food into her mouth—Cheryl wishes she had the time to do hand-over-hand feeding because she feels Katya would be feeding herself much sooner. Katya also continued to improve in reaching for, grasping of, and pulling things to herself—even holding items up and looking at them. Katya also helped her mother more during dressing and transfers. Cheryl could tell her to do a movement to help, such as bend her arm to dress, or roll into a ball so that Cheryl could carry her more easily, and she began doing as Cheryl asked and with less delay time. And Katya was smiling more when she could comply.

Katya's conscious presence and efforts to communicate have shown much improvement. She has more vocalizations and communicative interaction with her parents: She smiles or laughs after they speak, sings along with them, attempts new sounds, tries to make herself understood, and is very pleased when she succeeds. Eye contact has improved, and she is listening to and following conversations better.

The Dvoraks feel Katya is developing progressive understanding. She anticipates events (for example, she squeals and softens her hand to hold a spoon when she sees food); she responds more appropriately (laughing at funny things and smiling when praised); and she appears to be more focused, such as when she moves her head to look down at her food, as if thinking about what it is she's eating and how she might get it to her mouth.

That Katya can consciously initiate work on head control is new and very significant. Before stem cells, Katya's always held her head slumped onto her left shoulder and tried to lift it only when her parents dangled things of interest in front of her during physical therapy. Nor did she consciously use her head to look around at her environment. Now at six months post-treatment, she was articulating her head better and showing more interest in her environment.

With effort, the Dvoraks were able to raise the money for a second hUCSC infusion, which Katya received on August 9, 2004—her thirteenth birthday. Now, almost six months later, the Dvoraks are thrilled with Katya's expanding and deepening progress. The cognition they always suspected was there is surfacing, and they feel the stem cells are responsible for her gradually being able to "come out and play in the world more." A year and only two treatments after they started this journey, the Dvoraks are a household beginning to experience happiness for the first time. Aware of the saying that parents are only as happy as their most unhappy child, Cheryl feels that, in their case, happiness blossoms as Katya becomes a happier child in the face of all of her growing successes. Cheryl tries not to think of where Katya might be had they been able to swing more treatments, or a greater number of stem cells. She focuses on what is, and the successes they are all seeing and rejoicing in.

Within a month of Katya's second treatment with hUCSCs, Katya seemed to be demonstrating improved memory and thinking. She was more intent at listening, made very direct eye contact, had faster and more appropriate responses and an increased awareness of everything going on around her, and vocalized as if conversing. Though her parents still cannot discern exact phrases, they can hear more differentiated sounds, and Katya responds more immediately now when they speak to her. She does so with sounds, direct eye contact while moving lips and tongue, or words the Dvoraks can understand, such as "good morning" and "Mom:" followed by a "sentence." Before, their interactions with Katya were not distinct. She would stare blankly or just take a very long time to attempt to respond to people. Cheryl thinks she just couldn't process except with a lot of effort and time. Or her vocalizations seemed more random. Now the Dvoraks can converse with Katya, and feel she is definitely a party to what's going on. One caregiver stated: "She has a more normal laugh now—not those abrupt bursts." So now there is more control.

Head control continues to progress—Cheryl loves it when Katya constantly looks down at her food while eating. Because food has become such a positive stimulus for her, this is a time when one can really see her working at fine head movements—something never seen before! Also, her hand and arm work continue to improve. She now reaches out to hit a switch when asked (and smiles broadly while doing so) and is attempting to move/turn pages in books, as big a motivator as food. Her muscles are still very tight—she seems to have to tighten up to execute a movement, but she also seems more receptive to change: She listens to explanations of "please soften and relax," and Cheryl sees her thinking about this and shifting her body part in attempts to comply. After twelve years of tightening only, Cheryl considers this a miracle. The Dvoraks feel that more treatments will help her to practice and execute more and more fluid movements, through increased communication combined with her increased ability to carry out requests.

At one year since the Dvoraks began this journey, Katya is attempting and enjoying more physical skills, interacting with her parents more clearly, and is happier. She is creating new "Katya phrases": new combinations of sounds that resemble words and, at times, go on and on—like any person getting a point across—accompanied by intense eye gaze. When the Dvoraks speak to Katya, she immediately attempts a response of some kind in an effort to get them to understand: her mouth and tongue start moving, sounds come out, she looks hard at her parents (eye gaze before stem cells was mostly indirect).

Katya is having the best days in school she has ever had. Her physical therapist and aide report her willingness to do tasks that before stem cells she wouldn't tolerate, such as bearing weight for long periods of time in her gait trainer. When she sees her computer, she understands it is for communication. For example, when she arrives home with a "message from school" on it, she gets very excited when her parents turn it on, extends her hand to push the switch, and smiles throughout the message. She is more social and happy at school. She gets excited when her peers enter the room and relates to them more. The Dvoraks always believed that Katya was a people person, because she seemed to be calm and at peace around her friends, but now her parents are seeing more open displays of camaraderie in her smiles, vocalization/conversations, and eye contact with friends.

Eye contact is greatly improved: she can now look directly into Cheryl's eyes from way across the room as well as during their conversations. Katya wants to converse with the Dvoraks, wants to help, and is pleased when Cheryl thanks her for helping. She delights in being part of whatever is going on—after so many years of uncertainty about where she was, the Dvoraks are now experiencing interactions with their daughter! This is so exciting for them. All Cheryl can think of is when they will be able to get her next treatment so that they can continue to see her blossom.

There is so much more to look forward to: more motivation on Katya's part in initiating activities, clearer speech, more refined movements leading to self-feeding, taking steps, and everything else. Just in the last month Katya has been trying to roll over on her own. She deftly picks up her head, pulls her arms and legs forward into a ball, and rolls to the left with a big smile. She isn't completing it yet, but is certainly demonstrating the will to do so.

Cheryl's dream is for Katya to be able to have infusions every three months, or infusions of more stem cells per treatment, because the conscious and physical results Cheryl sees are dramatic. For someone as physically challenged as Katya, Cheryl feels certain more is better at this point. Katya is taking pride in her accomplishments and successes, which are considerable for just one year, and the Dvoraks can believe that Katya has the potential to do progressively more for herself, whereas before stem-cell treatment, potential wasn't in sight. Katya is also a more social and happy person who smiles and laughs a lot—the change is like gold from dross.

Like any parent, Cheryl hopes to direct her teenager in learning to guide herself through life, which implies a will and eagerness to take the wheel. Pre-stem cells, Cheryl saw no possibility of reaching this goal. A year later, she sees a spark of independent life in Katya's responses and abilities and more determination in her eyes. The Dvoraks have held on to a vision for Katya for twelve years. Now it seems possible she will someday share her own vision with them.

Postscript: Katya received her third hUCSC treatment on August 18, 2005, in Mexico. (The treatment was given by Fernando Ramirez, M.D.)

STROKE

When blood flow in the brain is obstructed due to a clogged blood vessel, a blood clot, or a weakened blood vessel that ruptures, a person is said to have had a stroke. This is a rather serious condition that affects 700,000 Americans annually and is the third leading cause of death in adults. About 29 percent of patients die within one year following a stroke; this figure rises in people age sixty-five and older. When blood flow to the brain is obstructed for any reason, this vital organ suffers a loss of energy and becomes injured. If the reduction in blood flow is sustained, brain tissue in the injured area dies or works poorly. This can bring about changes in speech, behavior, thought patterns, memory, and even permanent brain damage or death.

There are two types of stroke: ischemic stroke and hemorrhagic stroke. These are discussed below.

Ischemic Stroke

The most common type of stroke is an ischemic stroke. It occurs when a blood vessel clogs from within and reduces blood flow to the brain. Approximately 80 percent of all strokes are of this type. Generally, ischemic strokes result from an obstruction in a blood vessel, typically caused by a blood clot. These clots fall into two broad types: One is a cerebral thrombus, which refers to a blood clot that develops at the site of the clogged portion of a blood vessel. The other is a cerebral embolism, a term applied when a blood clot forms in a portion of the circulatory system outside the brain. Some of this clot then dislodges, enters the bloodstream, and winds up in blood vessels of the brain where it enters a vessel that is smaller than the clot. The clot then lodges in this small vessel and obstructs the flow of blood to a specific part of the brain, leading to a stroke.

Signs of Stroke

- *Sudden numbness or weakness of the face, arm or leg, especially on one side of the body.*
- *Sudden confusion, trouble speaking, or understanding.*
- *Sudden trouble seeing in one or both eyes.*
- *Sudden trouble walking, dizziness, loss of balance or coordination.*
- *Sudden, severe headache with no known cause.*

Source: American Stroke Association, a Division of American Heart Association, *http://www.strokeassociation.org/presenter.jhtml?identifier=1020*

One major cause of these types of clots is an irregular heartbeat called "atrial fibrillation." In atrial fibrillation, one of the two chambers (atria) of the heart goes into a kind of spasm that can lead to the formation of clots within the heart. These can then leave the heart and travel to the brain. These erratic heart spasms can be readily detected when a physician feels the patient's pulse. When atrial fibrillation is diagnosed, medications can effectively treat it or, in specific instances, the patient can undergo a surgical procedure that cures the condition. There are also many natural measures that help manage this condition, such as judicious use of magnesium along with the amino acid L-taurine.

Prior to having a major stroke, many people experience small or mini-strokes called "transient ischemic attacks" (TIAs). In a TIA, the blood supply to the brain is compromised for a short period of time with little or no signs afterward of permanent damage. The symptoms of a TIA may last from few minutes up to several hours.

Hemorrhagic Stroke

A hemorrhagic stroke occurs when a blood vessel ruptures, causing blood to leak into the brain. This type of stroke accounts for approximately 20 percent of all stroke cases. It happens when a weakened blood vessel in the brain ruptures and bleeds into the surrounding tissue. There are two types of weakened blood vessels that usually cause a hemorrhagic stroke: aneurysms and arteriovenous malformations (AVMs).

An aneurysm refers to a ballooning out of a weakened region of a blood vessel. If left untreated, an aneurysm will continue to weaken until it ruptures and bleeds into the brain.

An arteriovenous malformation (AVM) is a cluster of abnormally formed blood vessels in the brain, any one of which may rupture, causing bleeding into the brain.

Research scientists have used stem cells from human umbilical-cord blood on rats with strokes. They found that these human stem cells were not rejected nor did they cause any adverse effects; they entered the brain, survived, changed into cells with neuronal characteristics, and improved the neurological function of the paralyzed animals. Similar results are being reported in studies involving brain-injured humans.

The Thomas Christensen Story

We've all read or heard tell of people whose lives were turned upside down by the consequences of a single oversight or presumption. Many are young and risk takers by nature, who at some level harbor the illusion they are immortal—or at least temporarily immune from "paying the piper." This was pretty much the mindset of twenty-two-year-old aircraft mechanic Thomas Christensen during the summer of 1978. It was a mythic bubble that was about to burst.

On August 7, 1978, Christensen had his sights set on participating in a friend's wedding that was slated to take place that afternoon. Wanting to look his best, he hopped on his motorcycle and headed over to a nearby barbershop for a ritual "ear lowering." Since the trip from the barber to the wedding was a very short one and he wanted to keep his newly styled hair neat, Thomas decided to forgo wearing a helmet. The next thing he knew he was sliding in loose gravel at the top of a hill and heading for a light pole. The resulting crash left Thomas with a punctured lung, a broken collarbone, a right leg broken in three places below the knee, all his ribs in disarray; and he was in a comatose state that would drag on for twelve and a half weeks.

Though not expected to live, Thomas beat the odds and was thus dubbed "Miracle Boy" by his neurosurgeon. Miracle or not, the Thomas that emerged from the coma was light years away from his pre-accident state: He could not walk, talk, write, or even swallow. Although he could comprehend some of the signs in the hospital, and even recognize some family members who visited him, that was about it. It was on this foundation that Thomas and his doctors and therapists began the arduous task of rebuilding his life.

By the time Thomas left the hospital many months later, he could walk with a walker, handle routine self-care tasks like shaving, read and understand basic written materials, and speak (albeit slowly and with difficulty). His right side, which had been totally paralyzed following the accident, gradually recovered some function so that Thomas was able to once again write with his right hand and use his right leg. Walking and swimming helped strengthen and tone his body, but the overall weakness in Thomas's right side persisted.

Being a man of faith, Thomas held fast to the belief that the Almighty was not through with him and that good things would be coming his way. This steadfast belief helped Thomas surmount many hurdles including that of getting a driver's license—and eventually finding a wife, Judith, as well as a stepdaughter!

Sometimes one blessing leads to another, and this proved very true with Thomas and his stepdaughter. She had heard good things about the pioneering brain-repair work that was being done at the Brain Therapeutics Medical Clinic, and encouraged Thomas to see what they could do for him. He decided to try it and proceeded to undergo a series of treatments including hyperbaric oxygen, physical therapy, as well as other treatments. As a result, he began to walk on his own and to speak more clearly.

In December 2003, life took a decided downturn for Thomas when he fell for no apparent reason and found that his left side was paralyzed. Fortunately, a cleaning lady was present and was able to summon paramedics. By the time Thomas reached a local hospital, he was beginning to recover some ability to use his left side. The doctors did a CAT scan that indicated a blockage in blood vessels adjacent to the area of his original injury. An MRI proved inconclusive, leading Thomas's physicians to conclude that he had not had a stroke, but a "vascular incident." Later on an experienced neuro-rehab physician would conclude that a vascular blockage had occurred due to a sinus infection. Thomas was told to take aspirin to prevent future clots from forming and blocking a blood vessel in his brain, and was turned over to physical therapists who would try to help ameliorate his partial paralysis.

Thomas and his wife were not exactly satisfied with the pace of recovery afforded by the treatments he was receiving, so they began looking for more promising, science-based alternatives. It wasn't long before they discovered articles about the way that stem cells were being employed experimentally to treat neurological damage in both animals, and to a limited extent, humans. They were not especially keen on fetal or embryonic cells, having learned of the published studies indicating that these cells occasionally gave rise to tumors in animals. However, umbilical-cord stem cells looked very attractive—both in terms of safety and effectiveness in repairing brain-damaged rodents. And although many influential stem-cell researchers expressed doubts as to whether hUCSCs could bring about neurological restoration or regeneration in brain-damaged humans, the Christensens were not convinced; they were encountering numerous Internet articles reporting on significant clinical responses to hUCSC treatments in children and adults with conditions such as traumatic brain injury and cerebral palsy.

This investigative process led the Christensens to Dr. Ramirez's clinic, where Thomas received treatment on March 10, 2004. In the weeks that followed, many improvements began to surface: The fifth finger on Thomas's left hand, which had curled up following his vascular incident, straightened out. He was also able to speak more rapidly now than prior to treatment, and his progress with a walker prompted his physical therapist to comment that his post-stem-cell progress was his first real progress.

Today Thomas continues to get about with a walker and does various kinds of physical therapy. A heart problem that precipitated his stroke was uncovered early in 2005, and reparative surgery was done to prevent recurrences. The Christensens are now looking forward to Thomas's next hUCSC treatment.

AMYOTROPHIC LATERAL SCLEROSIS (ALS)

Amyotrophic lateral sclerosis (ALS), also called Lou Gehrig's disease, is a progressive disease characterized by the wasting away of certain nerve cells in the brain and spinal column called "motor neurons." Motor neurons control the muscles that facilitate movement, called "voluntary muscles."

Over a period of months or years, ALS sufferers experience increasing muscle weakness, an inability to control movement, and problems with speaking, swallowing, and breathing. However, the ability to think or reason remains intact. It does not produce abnormal sensations (tingling or numbness) or loss of sensation in the body. In short, the ALS patient's body shuts down, while the brain remains unimpaired. The famed University of Cambridge physicist Steven Hawking has ALS—in his case, a slowly progressive variant of the disease that has taken its toll on the great man's life for more than thirty years.

In the United States and most other parts of the world, one to two out of every 100,000 people develop ALS each year; men are affected slightly more often than women. Although ALS may occur at any age, it is most common in middle-aged and older adults.

The cause of ALS is unknown, although approximately 5 to 10 percent of people with the condition have an inherited form of it. There may be other as of yet unrecognized causes too. For example, some physicians feel that Lyme disease may produce ALS or an ALS-like state. There are case histories of people diagnosed with ALS who were later diagnosed with Lyme disease, who were successfully treated for this infection, and who then went on to experience a return to normal or near-normal function.

One reason Lyme disease may be missed is that the regular laboratory tests that virtually all doctors rely on do not accurately zero in on the Lyme disease antibodies. Even the Centers for Disease Control (CDC) in Atlanta apparently do not utilize the more reliable forms of testing, but instead those that tend to generate both false positives and false negatives. People with Lyme disease who get treatment in the form of antibiotics sometimes experience a nasty disease "die off" response known as a "Herxheimer reaction." Some also experience an overgrowth of yeast in their bodies that generates compounds known as mycotoxins, which can make ALS symptoms worse. After a course of antibiotic or antifungal therapy, many appear to go on to experience notable improvement in their condition.

Many doctors are also now performing in-depth analyses of the stool of ALS patients to see what kinds of bacteria, yeast, parasites, and so on they might be harboring, as well as performing a visual examination of the intestines for signs of inflammation. Some are also doing tests to see whether the patient is producing adequate hydrochloric acid (stomach acid), is digesting fats and proteins well, and has adequate amounts of short-chain fatty acids, which are essential to the structural integrity of the intestinal walls.

There are at least 400 different kinds of bacteria, yeast, viruses, and mycoplasmas that can inhabit the various regions of the intestine. In these regions, yeast and organisms that thrive in low or non-oxygen environments flourish; their growth can be encouraged by consumption of various sugars. When these organisms are deprived of food or killed off with antibiotics, they release or generate toxic compounds that can get through a damaged intestinal wall and affect the nervous system. This can make symptoms worse for some patients with various neurological diseases and conditions such as ALS.

These organisms can also cause the body to churn out a specific enzyme called "metalloproteinase-9" (MMP-9), which plays many roles in the human body. For one thing, it can weaken the intestinal wall, as well as the blood-brain barrier, and thus makes it more likely that noxious compounds can get through. This enzyme is also made and utilized by cancer cells to aid the spread of cancer throughout the human body. However, MMP-9 is also secreted by hUCSCs and plays a role in their ability to travel about the body and engraft. This being the case, the trick then is to reduce MMP-9 in body sites where it may interfere with hUCSC activity, but not interfere with the stem cell's ability to secrete MMP. In most instances, doctors try to heal up the dysbiotic gut (overgrowth of fungi or "bad" bacteria in the gut), which basically shuts down the inappropriate production of MMP-9 there. They also sometimes use compounds that inhibit MMP-9 in the gut and elsewhere. Among these are cinnamon (*Cinnamomum cassia*), green tea, and turmeric root. Amino acid combinations such as L-arginine, L-lysine, and L-proline, along with vitamin C and green tea extract, as well as high dose pancreatic enzyme therapy have been shown to inhibit the production of MMP-9. Then, after the gut is healed and the systemic or circulating MMP-9 is reduced, the MMP inhibitors are stopped and hUCSCs are introduced into the patient's body. The cells can then secrete MMP-9 normally without encountering conditions or substances that interfere with it or them.

Currently, there is no cure for ALS. However, many physicians advocate identifying as many underlying and contributory causes as possible and then dealing with them, since they believe this treatment approach will help retard the progression of ALS. In Mexico and other countries, some doctors are now trying to boost MMP-9 in stem cells and concomitantly inhibit substances that specifically interfere with MMP-9 production or its activity (such as a group of proteins called "tissue inhibitors of matrix metalloproteinases" or TIMPs), and are then treating patients with human umbilical-cord stem cells. This approach appears to slow disease progression in some instances, probably by prolonging the survival of motor neurons. However, proving that this approach works will require a great deal more data garnered from the responses of the ALS patients being treated.

The Lana McMillan Story

Life, we are told, can turn on a dime. Lana McMillan discovered how true this is when a freak injury during 1994 revealed that beneath the surface of apparent good health all was not quite right. Though she made what seemed to be a full recovery from her injury, she noticed that she was unable to walk as effortlessly as she could before it. As she put it, ". . . there seemed to be an issue with my ability to lift my right leg" and she began limping. She drew hope and consolation, however, from the fact that some days were better than others, with stretches of time when she appeared to walk normally.

Limping continued to overshadow Lana's life, and in 1996, she decided to seek medical assistance. In quick succession, she saw a general practitioner, an orthopedic specialist, and a neurologist. The GP and orthopedic specialist found nothing alarming. The neurologist, however, noted the absence of a right knee-jerk reflex, despite repeated tests. Finally, the doctor tried Lana's left knee, which produced the appropriate response.

This neurologist immediately referred Lana to other medical specialists in neurology. Among the tests she underwent were x-rays, EMGs (muscle performance evaluation tests), MRIs (magnetic resonance imaging), and blood tests. This battery of tests led her doctors to attribute Lana's physical woes to a compressed spinal disc in the lower back (L5–S1 level). The recommended solution: A surgical repair procedure called a laminectomy—that is, surgical removal of part of a vertebra.

Lana spent an unsuccessful year and half in physical therapy, hoping to avoid surgery. In 1999, she had the laminectomy procedure her physicians had originally suggested, followed by another year and a half of physical therapy, with some apparent improvement. Lana was now able to use weight-lifting exercise machines, incrementally increasing the weight and doing more repetitions over time. She also did demanding exercises in a pool. However, over time, she continued to limp.

From January 2001 on, Lana was frustrated to find herself dependent on a walker. Another round of consultations and the familiar litany of tests—EMGs, MRIs, a myelogram, and blood tests—were to no avail. Lana also began having problems with her right arm and hand. Many of her doctors acknowledged the presence of a problem but had no idea what was wrong with her.

On her neurologist's recommendation, she visited the University of Miami Medical Center (UM) where she got the impression the examining doctor was picking up on a fairly severe neurological problem, but did not acknowledge it. He reviewed her medical records in detail and did some cursory tests, including the knee-reflex test. On subsequent visits, he performed an EMG, an MRI (including a brain MRI that she had not previously), and more blood tests. He concluded that she appeared to have a degenerative spinal-cord disease. Her condition was diagnosed in January 2003 as amyotrophic lateral sclerosis (ALS).

Lana's initial response was one of shock, anger, and then depression. For the better part of the next month, she withheld any mention of the diagnosis when talking to family and close friends; then, she relented and began divulging her heart-rending situation.

By this time, her physical condition had deteriorated; she was unable to rise from a seated position without some type of assistance. Often, she chose seats that were high enough to wiggle into, leaving her feet dangling above the floor. When she was ready to stand, she would scoot forward and wiggle off the chair into a standing position; chairs with arms allowed Lana to push herself out and then stand. Sadly, her legs alone were no longer strong enough to lift her up to a standing position.

On the day she was diagnosed, Lana was also introduced to the Kessenich Family MDA ALS Center and was given a prescription for Rilutek and an appointment for a follow-up session. The Kessenich Family MDA ALS Center is a multidimensional support and advanced research center into the cause and cure of ALS. It provides a high level of care for ALS patients and their families—from the time of diagnosis throughout the course of the disease—assisting them in the management of the disease by providing resources such as physical therapy, occupational therapy, speech therapy, communication, respiratory therapy, transportation, equipment, nutrition counseling, nursing services, lung and GI-tract medical services, and psychological support. The center also organizes and supervises ALS support groups, conducts clinical trials, and keeps patients informed of the latest developments related to ALS.

The center sent Lana home with a wealth of ALS literature. She immediately set about researching ALS through personal contacts, pamphlets, library visits, and Internet surfing. After reading other people's stories and talking with them, she also began taking nutritional supplements. After failing to qualify for a Mayo Clinic study because she'd had ALS symptoms for too long, Lana learned that, for the same reason, she could not participate in any trials conducted by the Kessenich Family MDA ALS Center. These rejections sparked a quest to find a treatment that was more aggressive and promising than the Rilutek and nutritional supplements she was already taking.

One such treatment was calcium EAP (ethanolamine-phosphate), developed by the late German physician Dr. Hans Nieper. Although this therapy is not available through an IV or an injection in the

United States, Lana succeeded in finding a medical doctor who was willing to help her continue Dr. Nieper's calcium EAP regimen stateside. Although this approach was originally developed for people with remitting relapsing multiple sclerosis, Dr. Nieper reported seeing some degree of success in treating ALS patients with calcium EAP.

During this time, Lana read Jim Haverlock's story on the Internet and wrote him a letter (see pages 41–44). Jim responded, telling Lana of the benefits he had received from calcium EAP, and told her that he was now onto something that looked far better: stem-cell therapy. Jim graciously provided Lana with the information she needed to research stem-cell therapy for herself.

On Jim's recommendation, Lana contacted Dr. Anthony G. Payne at the Steenblock Research Institute in California and learned about treatments being provided at various foreign clinics; these were a bit too costly for Lana. However, there was one firm called BioMark International that was offering to help patients get treated with three-million CD34 umbilical-cord stem cells as part of a Canadian pilot study. Participants paid for their airfare to Vancouver, their hotel expenses, and $10,000 for the cost of the cells. Lana opted to take this route.

In Vancouver, Lana's treatment consisted of two separate subcutaneous injections into two different areas of the abdominal region above and near her stomach.

Almost immediately, Lana found it easier (though not easy) to stand from a seated position and she could also stand from her power chair (or toilet) on the first try. Prior to stem-cell therapy, it had taken multiple attempts to stand from either.

Lana also experienced an upsurge in her energy level. She was much less tired and lethargic than she had been. Friends commented on how much better she looked and noted that her skin appeared much softer and healthier.

Shortly afterward, Lana noted the disappearance of an odd tingling she had been experiencing each morning in her right arm. Persistent cramps and pains in her right forearm were also gone. She now found that she could cut up her food more easily, and could hold a glass without dropping it. (Prior to stem-cell therapy, Lana could hardly cut up a waffle or refrain from dropping everything she tried to hold.)

Lana also found it easier to wiggle the toes on her right foot, as well as to extend the foot farther out in front of her from a seated position. She noticed that a long-standing twitching in her legs and arms was virtually gone.

Lana at first thought she might be experiencing the placebo effect. But the improvements persisted, and she did not regress, except briefly during the eighth or ninth week.

More than six months have elapsed since Lana received umbilical-cord stem cells, and nearly all the improvements that appeared during the first month remain. To whit: It is easier to stand; she has more vim and vigor; there are no cramps or pains in her right forearm; her right arm does not go to sleep when she wakes up; it is easier to cut up food; and she isn't dropping things as often.

Lana adds, "You have to take the good with the bad," and yes, some things have continued to decline. She has more difficulty extending her right arm or raising it over her head. When seated, she cannot put her right leg out as far as she could shortly after receiving stem cells. Turning over in bed has also become difficult, and it is getting harder to lift her right leg. Also, when Lana is lying down, she can barely move her right leg. Generally she has to move it by pushing her left leg against the right, or by using her arms to move it.

All in all, though, Lana is very happy she received the umbilical-cord stem cells. She has experienced definite improvement "and that for someone with ALS is saying a lot." To her way of thinking, the stem cells have bought her a little more time and improved the quality of her life. And she is thankful for that much.

Currently, Lana is seeking further stem-cell treatment. Since ALS is a progressive disease, she feels that she will probably require repeat treatments to sustain her improvements, and she hopes to regain some of the bodily functions she's lost to the disease. If Lana's goal is realized, then perhaps her affliction will become more manageable. Not cured by any means, but held at bay until medical science has a more effective approach to treating ALS.

TRAUMATIC BRAIN INJURY

Traumatic brain injury (TBI) or "head injury" occurs when a sudden trauma causes damage to the brain. This can result with the sudden impact of a person's head with an object, or when something penetrates the skull and enters the brain. TBIs that result in mild damage to the brain often result in such symptoms as headache, confusion, dizziness, lightheadedness, ringing in the ears, fatigue or lethargy, sleep disturbances, behavioral or mood changes, and difficulties with memory, concentration, focus, or thinking. Moderate or severe TBI symptoms will often mirror those of the milder type, but may also include a headache that gets worse or does not fade out, convulsions or seizures, loss of coordination, trouble stirring from sleep, slurred speech, repeated vomiting or nausea, weakness or numbness in the extremities, and increased confusion, restlessness, or agitation.

For doctors, the most pressing concern when it comes to a fresh TBI is to insure that a proper oxygen supply reaches the brain and the rest of the body, along with maintaining adequate blood flow, and keeping blood pressure normalized. About half of all TBI patients require surgical intervention to remove or repair ruptured blood vessels or brain tissue.

Generally speaking, the degree of disability arising from a TBI depends upon the location and severity of the injury, and the age and general health of the individual. TBIs frequently result in problems with cognition (thinking, memory, and reasoning); one's sense of sight, hearing, touch, taste, and smell; communication (expression and understanding); and conduct or mental health. More serious head injuries may result in stupor, an unresponsive state, though the individual can be aroused briefly by sharp pain; coma, in which an individual is totally unconscious, unresponsive, unaware, and can't be roused; a vegetative state, in which a sufferer is unconscious and unaware of his or her surroundings, but continues to have a sleep-wake cycle and periods of alertness; and a persistent vegetative state (PVS), in which an individual remains in a vegetative state for more than a month.

The Austin Wade Story

Helen's son, Austin Wade, was born at home in a water tub on September 7, 2004. It was a beautiful birth, and he seemed perfect. Then on October 15, 2004, the Wade's world crashed. Austin had a severe bleed on his brain and was rushed into emergency brain surgery. The bleed was so massive that part of Austin's brain emerged when the surgical team went in to stop the bleeding. The surgeons had to remove Austin's left bone flap because they knew his brain would continue to swell. Austin spent two weeks in intensive care and came home with the bone flap extending from his head.

The bleed on Austin's brain had occurred because he was not given a vitamin K shot at birth. With a simple vitamin K shot, he would be a healthy, happy child today. In December 2004, Austin had his second surgery and the bone in his head was replaced. The swelling on his brain had gone down. But doctors gave the Wades dire news. When the swelling went down, his whole brain sustained massive damage. The doctors told the Wades that Austin would be mentally retarded, but could not tell them to what extent.

Austin does not visually track objects, leading doctors to believe that he is cortically blind. At ten months old, he does not roll over, cannot sit unassisted, and cannot crawl or move like most babies. He can move his body, however, and is able to breathe and nurse. He weighs quite a bit more than he should (at ten months old, Austin weighs thirty-one pounds), and the Wades are waiting for hormone test results to find out if something is causing his extreme weight.

On May 23, 2005, Austin received an injection of umbilical-cord stem cells. Since then, the Wades have seen some improvements, the biggest of which is that he has started to laugh. He is also cooing more and is playing with his left hand, in which he has more coordination, more frequently. And Austin's napping pattern has improved. Before stem cells, his naps were from five to fifteen minutes; now, he will often sleep for a half hour to an hour at a time during the day. He manages to sleep through the night, which he'd been doing since the bone flap was replaced in his head.

Responses to hUCSC Therapy by Disease or Condition

One of the things scientists try to figure out when a new type of biologic therapy or treatment is being assessed is how various diseases or conditions respond to it. After more than two and a half years of accruing information—doctor/patient/caregiver feedback and the results of standardized medical assessment tests—researchers at Steenblock Research Institute have come up with a general, though admittedly tentative, breakdown of how well or poorly various conditions respond to hUCSC therapy. Here are their findings:

Good Responders

- *Cerebral palsy in children and young adults*

- *Various eye diseases and conditions, including diabetic retinopathy*

- *Acute stroke and other circulatory problems that occurred recently*

Marginal Responders

- *Multiple sclerosis (various types, especially advanced); improvements occur, but some are typically lost to disease progression*

- *Early-stage amyotrophic lateral sclerosis (ALS)*

Poor Responders

- *Chronic stroke (acute stroke refers to the hours and first two or three days following a stroke. The period after the acute phase is referred to as "chronic.")*

- *Amyotrophic lateral sclerosis—middle and later stages especially.*

Austin seems to look at objects more, and people have told Helen that he seems more alert. The Wades are looking forward to Austin's next stem-cell treatment. They feel his improvements are substantial enough to warrant more stem-cell treatments and are excited about the future and feel blessed to be able to give their little boy a fighting chance to live a quality life.

CONCLUSION

If one thinks of the human body as a house, then surely stem cells qualify as being integral members of its repair and restoration (R&R) crew. However, when the house is in too great a state of disrepair or is falling apart faster than the R&R crew can keep up with it, then help is needed from outside sources. Depending on the cause of the disrepair, hUCSCs can be one of these sources. However, it helps to get as much of the debris cleared out as possible before sending in the hUCSC team.

Since 2003, researchers at Steenblock Research Institute have been implementing and assessing various ways to "clear out the debris," as well as to make sure the R&R team (hUCSCs) can get to target tissues or organs and then do their job. Along the way, the SRI staff has accumulated and analyzed response data on more than 100 people treated with hUCSCs for a wide variety of health challenges. So far, people with conditions such as cerebral palsy, traumatic brain injury (TBI), diabetic neuropathy, diabetic retinopathy, macular degeneration, acute stroke, and early to mid-stage multiple sclerosis and ALS have shown the greatest overall benefit. Preliminary indications are that arthritis also responds well to hUCSC treatment. On the flipside, chronic stroke, advanced multiple sclerosis and ALS, Alzheimer's disease, and some forms of chronic obstructive pulmonary disease do not appear to improve greatly. Still unknown is how well such widespread human maladies as Parkinson's disease and various kinds of kidney disease will respond to IV-infused or implanted hUCSCs, although many researchers feel there is great potential for improvement using cord-blood stem cells.

CHAPTER 5

Questions and Answers on Umbilical-Cord Stem-Cell Therapy

S teenblock Research Institute has been tracking and analyzing patient responses to human umbilical-cord stem-cell therapy carried out in Mexico since early 2003. During this time, many questions have been posed by laypeople, reporters, and a good many physicians and scientists concerning human umbilical-cord stem cells, their nature, therapeutic use, safety, and effectiveness. These questions were systematically collected and responses were formulated by researchers at SRI. This chapter contains the most frequently asked questions.

Q. Is umbilical-cord stem-cell therapy safe?

A. Physicians in the United States have used stem-cell-rich cord-blood infusions to treat various hematopoietic (blood-related) diseases for about forty years. In the majority of cases, patients who have received these infusions have not developed stem-cell-related post-treatment diseases or cancers. Members of the National Institutes of Health (NIH) stated in 2003 that they see no cases of cancer or other health threats arising from stem-cell therapy. Moreover, researchers at the Steenblock Research Institute have yet to encounter a single instance of rejection in patients who have received pure umbilical-cord progenitor (stem) cells—housed in a liquid medium virtually free of added growth factors. This suggests that umbilical-cord stem-cell therapy is very safe.

Q. How quickly do stem-cell recipients see results?

A. Many physicians and researchers have observed and noted major improvements in patients within the first three or four months after stem-cell therapy, with less pronounced changes thereafter. There are numerous reports of benefits from the therapy in as little as twenty-four hours after treatment; however, because the stem cells don't engraft and proliferate this soon, these benefits probably result from the body's production of growth factors and specific compounds in response to the presence of the cells.

While improvements typically take place within three or four months, there are cases where improvement may occur later. For example, an eighty-three-year-old retired banker from Boston had an infusion of umbilical-cord stem cells for the express purpose of regaining some of the depth perception he'd lost in one eye after a stroke—mainly so he could get back out on the golf course! This fellow was slow to respond and experienced only modest improvements in his vision during the first two to three months after the treatment. But then, over the next six months, he gradually recovered enough of his vision to discern large objects.

Q. How much does stem-cell therapy cost? What about pre- and post-treatments?

A. The costs for hUCSC treatments vary widely, but a ballpark range for a single stem-cell treatment is $8,000 to $25,000. Pre- and post-treatment care such as testing for heavy metals and gut dysbiosis (where suspected), use of intermittent hypoxia therapy to create conditions in the body stem cells favor, treatment with external counterpulsation therapy to get blood vessels in injured but healed-over areas to once again produce signals such as VEGF (vascular endothelial growth factor) that attract stem cells, physician monitoring following treatment, and so on can run as much as $6,000 to $10,000 or more. It should be noted that Dr. Fernando Ramirez (Tijuana, Mexico) charges $8,000 per hUCSC treatment (~2.0 million hUCSCs, Fall 2005). (See the Resources section.)

Q. Do insurance companies cover umbilical-cord stem-cell therapy?

A. Since stem-cell therapy is currently experimental and unproved, the insurance industry has no obligation to recognize it as a reimbursable form of medical therapy. There is, however, at least one approved form: cord-blood infusions for certain blood-borne disorders such as leukemia following destruction of bone marrow by radiation and/or chemotherapy.

Q. Is pre-treatment necessary? What about post-treatment?

A. Children with neurological challenges such as cerebral palsy and traumatic brain injury (TBI) appear to respond well without any pre- or post-treatments. This is likely due to the strong biochemical signals being given off by the parts of their nervous system that are damaged or inflamed. And indeed, a number of animal and some published human studies have found inflammatory compounds being generated in damaged brains such as stromal-derived growth factor-alpha (SDF-alpha). SDF-alpha has been shown to attract stem cells to damaged or inflamed brain tissue like a "homing beacon" by researchers such as Evan Snyder, M.D., Ph.D., at the Burnham Institute in La Jolla, California.

People with recent injuries or conditions, as well as those with active diseases, also appear to benefit without much in the way of any pre- or post-treatments geared to "amplify" these signals. However, in patients with old wounds or damage, as well as those with diseases that do not involve inflammation, there is a need to get the organ or tissues that need repair or regeneration to produce stem-cell homing signals such as stromal-derived growth factor-alpha. In many instances, these signals can be elicited from healed-over tissues by using a hormone such as erythropoietin, as well as by application of medical technologies that tend to "tweak" tissues to get them to generate stem-cell attractant signals. Among these are external counterpulsation and intermittent hypoxia.

Counterpulsation involves wrapping huge inflatable cuffs around the abdomen and lower extremities. These cuffs are hooked up to an air compressor–computer device that inflates the cuffs each time the heart rests between beats. This process sends blood racing back toward the heart and brain. Such gentle pressure, it is felt, appears to coax healed-over tissue to once again begin churning out stem-cell-attracting biochemical signals. Intermittent hypoxia involves breathing oxygen through a mask at levels that are gradually lowered from normal to that of air found at higher elevations. This is akin to gradually climbing a mountain. This reduction in body-wide oxygen causes tissues or organs that were previously, or are currently, injured or diseased to begin producing biochemical compounds that tend to attract stem cells.

Q. Why do so many doctors "in the know" recommend umbilical-cord blood rather than embryonic or fetal stem cells?

A. Quality control and assurance is a major issue with so-called embryonic stem-cell therapy abroad. The cells being used apparently come from aborted fetuses. When questioned about the quality control and assurance used to ensure that the cells they advertise are actually more than just a hodgepodge from fetal tissue, those who use embryonic stem cells usually try to dodge the question or promise documentation but never send it. None of the representatives or medical directors involved in so-called embryonic stem-cell therapy who were contacted by the authors of this book was willing to provide specific quality control and assurance certificates of analysis or of any related material.

The umbilical-cord stem cells utilized by the clinics cited in this book, on the other hand, are processed using the very highest standards and state-of-the-art technology available. The cord blood itself is collected only from healthy mothers who give birth to full-term, normal, healthy babies, and is then screened for all major communicable diseases like HIV, hepatitis A, B, and C, and cytomegalovirus. At this stage, blood that is free of disease-causing viruses and such is sent to the lab where skilled technicians use special technology to separate various subtypes of hUCSCs—for example those bearing CD factors such as 133, 44, and 45 (see the inset "What Do the "CD" and "+" and "–" Mean?" on page 15). These stem cells are then grown in a brew of nutrients and growth factors that is free of any animal protein or compounds. After peak growth (expansion in numbers) is reached, the stem cells are placed in vials in amounts typically ranging from 1.5 to 3 million stem cells, and are then frozen in liquid nitrogen and stored. (Certificates of analysis are furnished to researchers and research-oriented physicians by the labs where the umbilical-cord-blood stem cells are produced.)

With regard to safety, it is important to keep in mind that embryonic stem cells have been used for less than a decade and mostly by scientists doing research in lab animals. No one can be absolutely certain of what secondary diseases or cancers may arise twenty years or so down the line as a result of the therapy. Lab studies have repeatedly shown that embryonic stem cells can form tumors when injected into lab animals. And, according to a confidential source in the European Union (EU), there are a few case histories of human embryonic stem-cell recipients in Portugal and elsewhere who developed cancer after their treatment. On the other hand, cord blood and the stem cells it contains have been used for more than forty years with virtually no secondary diseases or cancers as a result.

Q. *Are there side effects or risks associated with umbilical-cord stem-cell therapy?*

A. In the more than 100 cases being tracked by the staff of the Steenblock Research Institute, the only notable side effects have been fatigue that lasted for anywhere from a few hours to a few days or, conversely, heightened energy that typically ran its course in a few days. There have been instances of allergic reactions, but these were traced to an iodine-based topical antiseptic that was used prior to the stem-cell treatment. (These problems vanished once the use of this antiseptic was discontinued.) There have been reports of patients expe-

About the Children Needing a Miracle Foundation

Children Needing A Miracle Foundation (CNMF) is nonprofit organization that was set up specifically to help pay all or part of the cost of a stem-cell treatment for children from families who cannot afford the cost. You can visit the foundation on the Internet at www.childrenneedingamiracle foundation.com.

From the CNMF website:

Children Needing a Miracle Foundation was founded by the very talented and internationally renowned speaker and author, Kevin Hogan, Psy.D., out of his remarkable kindness and compassion for severely injured children.

Dr. Hogan directs Children Needing a Miracle Foundation to fulfill the mission he envisioned:

The mission for Children Needing a Miracle Foundation is to provide funding for the treatment of children who currently can't be helped by mainstream medicine.

CNMF will help qualifying children through funding for experimental and research treatments as well as providing funding for devices to enhance the quality of life of children who cannot be helped even through experimental means.

This includes helping severely brain and spine injured children needing a miracle recovery.

Treatments have been shown to aid in the recovery process for these children. CNMF also plans to give high priority to providing funds for umbilical cord stem cell therapy to children who are recommended for this procedure by a qualified physician with extensive training in this specialty.

Those wishing to make a tax deductible donation are encouraged to do so and should make checks payable to "Children Needing a Miracle Foundation" and mail them to 690 N. Farmersville Blvd, Farmersville, CA 93223.

Note: The authors of this book do not have any financial or other interest in the CNMF and do not benefit in any way whatsoever from its operation, nor does Steenblock Research Institute or Brain Therapeutics Medical Clinic.

riencing muscle twitches called "fasiculations" in response to the growth factors in umbilical-cord stem-cell vials coming from specific labs. This was not found to be true of hUCSC material from labs that diluted or washed out these growth factors.

So, overall, the risks appear to be negligible. The decade's-old use of stem-cell-rich cord blood has basically established these cells as safe, and the paucity of adverse reactions underscores this.

Q. What is the current status of FDA approval for stem-cell treatments?

A. The FDA has not approved embryonic stem-cell treatments for any disease or condition. However, bone marrow and other sources of adult stem cells have been approved for about eighty-six diseases. And cord blood—but not pure umbilical-cord stem cells—is allowed by the FDA for certain hematopoietic diseases such as leukemia.

The National Institutes of Health (NIH) and private companies are funding research, but a great deal of the research is focused on working out the basic biology in lab animals, so progress is slow. And although several state governments have passed legislation to actively encourage stem-cell research, these laws do not mean that physicians in these states can give umbilical-cord blood or isolated stem cells to patients in need (outside of approved conditions or as part of government-sanctioned clinical trials). Federal law is supreme above state law, so even if a state were to pass a law permitting medical doctors and osteopathic physicians (D.O.) to give stem cells to their patients, this statute would surely be struck down at the federal level.

Q. Why is stem-cell therapy permitted in Mexico, Costa Rica, and other countries, but not in the United States or Canada?

A. In the United States, the FDA has a legal mandate to protect the medical consumer's health and welfare. Since *embryonic* stem-cell therapy is truly a "vast undiscovered country" in terms of efficacy and long-term safety, the FDA is careful to enforce restrictions and regulations that keep it confined to the lab or the research center until it has been proven safe and effective. The Canadian Health Ministry has a similar policy.

However, while it's true that embryonic stem cells have been used for a relatively short time, the same cannot be said of umbilical-cord blood-derived stem cells. Stem-cell-rich cord blood has been used to treat hematopoietic diseases for more than forty years with virtually no secondary illnesses or complications. This alone shows the utility and safety of umbilical-cord stem cells. But even so, FDA regulations allow little latitude in their use except for treatment of approved conditions or in experiments that meet stringent criteria. Interestingly, the FDA has recently shown a willingness to allow the use of cord blood to treat neurological disease such as ALS and other intractable illnesses and conditions on a case-by-case basis. Still, the basic prohibition on open use of umbilical-cord stem cells or cord blood at a physician's discretion holds sway overall.

Scientific and medical experts differ widely on the issue of forging ahead, at least in terms of allowing umbilical-cord stem-cell therapy to be used freely by doctors for non-hematopoietic conditions here in the United States. Critics favor waiting for a consensus to emerge from ongoing research. Others agree, but draw the line when it comes to diseases or conditions for which existing drugs and other treatments offer little in the way of relief or benefit. Since pure umbilical-cord stem cells appear to pose no credible threat of rejection or adverse side effects, and may positively impact many illnesses for which standard treatments offer little if any relief or improvement, there is a compelling argument for giving physicians the right to readily obtain and freely use them to address such conditions and illnesses.

Q. Prior to receiving stem-cell therapy in Mexico, Costa Rica, or elsewhere, can a person visit the treatment facility?

A. Most clinics encourage prospective patients to visit them prior to undergoing stem-cell therapy. Many people time their visit to the clinic to coincide with their medical workup and pre-stem-cell treatment preparations, if indicated or desired. Others choose to visit the facility before making any decisions.

Q. Is hUCSC therapy guaranteed?

A. Umbilical-cord stem-cell therapy is not guaranteed. Aside from cord-blood treatments for leukemia and a handful of bloodborne diseases and conditions, it is still an experimental therapy and has not yet been scientifically proven effective for any given condition or disease. There are many factors that influence a patient's response to umbilical-cord stem cells, including age; genetics; the type, nature, and severity of the health condition; and nutritional status. Also, patients vary widely in terms of their compliance with pre- and post-treatment guidelines, such as physical therapy, dietary and nutrition regimens, and proper use of medications.

With this said, many patients who have received umbilical-cord stem cells have reaped benefits and gains that exceed what they were able to attain on standard therapies and conventional medical treatments, virtually without regression or adverse effects. (Note, however, that patients with progressive diseases such as primary progressive multiple sclerosis and amyotrophic lateral sclerosis do lose ground gradually.) Interestingly, *some* of the functional gains in progressive MS patients who are being followed by Steenblock Research Institute have not been significantly compromised or eroded in the years following treatment.

Q. Can a person treated with hUCSCs receive post-treatment care in his or her home state or country of residence?

A. Depending on the particular case, the post-treatment care prescribed by most reputable clinics that offer hUCSC therapy can usually be handled through a patient's own primary-care physician. This includes follow-up evaluations and testing such as blood and urine analysis, plus specific tests including but not limited to various types of x-rays and brain scans like MRIs (magnetic resonance imaging), computer tomography (CT), measurement of electrical activity in the brain (electroencephalograms; EEG), assessing nutritional status and disease or condition response, and so forth.

Q. Can a certain diet enhance the success of stem-cell therapy?

A. Steenblock Research Institute has devoted considerable time and resources to exploring dietary influences on patient responses to stem-cell therapy. The diet the Institute recommends is structured and fairly restrictive in certain respects, especially in terms of eliminating foods and dietary supplements that have proven harmful to stem cells in laboratory experiments. SRI researchers admit that the diet is eperimental and that a "dietary mistake" is unlikely to severely compromise stem-cell therapy. But even so, many patients who adhered to the diet appear to have fared better than "disease-matched" patients who did not.

One of the planks in the Steenblock Research Institute diet program is for patients to limit consumption of common allergy-producing foods such as cereal gluten grains (wheat, rye, barley, and oats), soy, and cow's milk. These foods generate opioid-like compounds called "exorphins" in the body that appear to contribute to inflammatory processes that may hinder nerve repair, especially in people with diseases that are characterized by a great deal of neuroinflammation— such as, amyotrophic lateral sclerosis and multiple sclerosis.

Readers who would like additional information about the effects of grains on the body might want to read *Dangerous Grains: Why Gluten Cereal Grains May Be Hazardous to Your Health* by James Braly, M.D. and Ron Hoggan (Avery Publishing Group, 2002); or *The Paleodiet* by Loren Cordain, Ph.D. (Wiley, 2002).

CONCLUSION

Human umbilical-cord stem cells have proven to be very safe for human medical application. Tentative evidence garnered from patient responses to hUCSC therapy done in Mexico by researchers at Steenblock Research Institute indicate that these stem cells bring about improvements in many people with cerebral palsy, traumatic brain injury (TBI), diabetic retinopathy and neuropathy, acute stroke, and a multitude of other neurologic disorders and diseases. At present, one research-oriented clinical program exists in Mexico that offers patients treatment with hUCSCs that are certifiably free of the most common blood-transmitted diseases such as HIV and hepatitis A, B, and C, and at a cost that appears unmatched. Readers interested in learning more should check the Resource section.

CHAPTER 6

Dietary Considerations
Following Stem-Cell Therapy

T he role of diet and lifestyle in promoting stem-cell activity, or
conversely in hindering it, is largely uncharted territory. Studies have shown that foods such as papaya and pineapple contain compounds that actually interfere with a cell's ability to divide and
thrive (proliferation). But do these foods cause problems for newly
introduced hUCSCs in people? And, on the flip side, are there certain
foods that tend to promote cell proliferation, and therefore might
encourage the proliferation of hUCSCs administered to people? And
what about prolonged exposure to intense electromagnetic fields such
as one might encounter by being close to certain electronic devices?
Do these interfere with cell proliferation? How about the effect of
spending lengthy time in direct sunlight following a treatment, or
engaging in physically intense activities? What about exposure to
things that cause physical, mental, and emotional stress? And what
about the use of antibiotics and other drugs or nutritional or herbal
supplements? Can having a drink or a smoke interfere with hUCSC
engraftment or subsequent activity?

Although Chapter 3 addresses some of the information in this
chapter, diet and lifestyle are considered very important players in a
patient's response to hUCSC therapy. Therefore, this chapter revisits
some of the earlier information and provides more details and further
dietary considerations.

EFFECT OF ENVIRONMENT AND DIET ON CELL DIVISION AND GROWTH—WHAT DO WE KNOW?

Major online medical databases, such as PubMed (National Library of Medicine), contain all sorts of citations and abstracts from journal papers concerning how certain environmental and dietary factors can impede or conversely spur on cell division and growth. Many of these reports center on studies that exposed cells to various compounds or environmental influences in a lab dish, while other reports deal with studies on mice, rats, and other animal models. However, a few of the studies actually involve human subjects. Some directly and squarely tackle a compound or environmental factor that hindered or accelerated cell proliferation in people. Some scientists and researchers suggest that an influence seen in a lab dish would logically apply to animals and people. Not surprisingly, some studies contradict other studies. Until definitive, rigorous scientific assessments are done and a consensus emerges, many aspects of what kind of diet or lifestyle modifications patients need to make following treatment with stem cells remains an admittedly open question.

However, the unknowns and tentativeness of dietary and lifestyle influences on post-treatment hUCSC activity does not mean that a worthy guiding compass does not exist. In fact, Dr. Fernando Ramirez, who was involved in transplanting animal cells and tissues into suitable human recipients for several decades prior to commencing work with hUCSCs, has keenly noted many dietary factors that tend to decrease a person's likelihood of a favorable outcome from these treatments. For example, red meat consumed during the first twelve days or so following transplants and infusions appears to decrease the kind and degree of clinical benefit patients reap (compared with those who refrain from consuming read meat altogether during this period). This may be related to the presence of specific compounds in cooked beef that tend to interfere with cell proliferation, such as oxidized fatty acids.

Dr. Ramirez and others involved in his program—including researchers who provide technical support at Steenblock Research Institute—began to systematically pool their insights, and observations, and material gleamed from the scientific record in 2003. From this information, a set of dietary and lifestyle guidelines was fashioned. During the ensuing years, these guidelines have been modified in light of new information coming in from published studies, as well as patient response data. Like many tools in medicine, this approach involves an interweaving of art and science, as much a process as an end in itself.

The post-hUCSC treatment program that has emerged is predicated on the *nature of human nature itself*—which is to say, what we as a species have evolved to thrive on in terms of diet and lifestyle. Evidence is steadily accruing to indicate that we as a species do better in terms of overall health and fitness when we live and eat in accordance with evolved patterns that go back millions of years; that we begin to develop certain chronic illnesses and conditions when we deviate significantly from these patterns, as has been the case since grains and cereals were domesticated and then increasingly consumed by people, beginning some 10,000 years ago.

Fossil evidence indicates that certain maladies increased in almost lock-step fashion with the corresponding increase in grain and cereal consumption as well as reliance on domesticated cattle and so on. Cereals and grains, for example, contain compounds called phytates that limit mineral absorption and can thus favor calcium loss, and thus, compromise bone function. Then, too, lipids (fats) from domesticated animal sources tend to contain a ratio of healthy to unhealthy fats that is out-of-kilter with what is found in wild game. This appears to be a major contributor to the ensuing increase in the incidence of coronary artery disease in the industrialized West. And there is a body of evidence that indicates that we evolved to thrive on a high intake of potassium and a low intake of sodium, and a dietary influx of calcium to magnesium of 1:1. In cultures where sodium is high and potassium is low, there are typically a great many people with sodium sensitive/triggered high blood pressure. And in settings where calcium intake is very high but magnesium is low, some folks appear to respond to this physiological imbalance by developing osteoporosis or hardening of the arteries.

The health-eroding consequences of these "dysnutritional" trends are being increasingly born out by studies done on archaeological human remains from every corner of the world; studies that demonstrate an increased evidence of poorer dental health, iron-deficiency anemia, infection and bone loss from the advent of agriculture onward.

HIGHLIGHTS OF THE POST-HUCSC TREATMENT DIET AND LIFESTYLE PROGRAM

During the first thirty days following a treatment with hUCSCs, the focus is limiting or removing anything that might tend to inhibit stem-cell proliferation or activity, while concomitantly introducing measures that support this process. The post-hUCSC treatment diet and lifestyle regimen that is recommended for patients who are part of the Ramirez program eliminates red meat, certain fruits and other foods for a short period of time, while allowing a nutrient-rich diet that consists of roughly 70 percent complex carbohydrates (vegetables and certain fruits) and 30 percent protein and healthy fats. The basic dietary pattern is consistent with that of our pre-agricultural, Paleolithic or "Stone-Age" ancestors, who ate no grains or cereals, ate game meat and fish that sported a healthy ratio of fats (omega-3 to omega-6 fatty acids), and did not consume milk in any form after weaning from their mother's breast milk.

Factors That May Inhibit Stem-Cell Growth and Thus Need to Be Avoided

- Close, prolonged exposure to high-intensity household and environmental electromagnetic fields, including poorly shielded cell phones, high-power electrical lines, television, and computers during the first day or so following treatment. These could potentially increase oxidative stress (cell-damaging free-radical production) and thus inhibit stem-cell proliferation.

- No papaya, pineapple, onions, garlic, ginger, apples, berries (such as cranberries, raspberries, blueberries, and blackberries), citrus fruits, honey, beer (hops), red wine, cauliflower, broccoli, Brussels sprouts, and almonds. These foods contain antiproliferative compounds and thus may interfere with stem-cell proliferation. This restriction applies for the first two weeks following stem-cell therapy, when hUCSCs are most likely to be finding a biological home, engrafting, and proliferating.

- No alcohol for at least six months following stem-cell therapy. It inhibits nerve growth factor and is toxic to new nerve-cell growth.

- No herbs or herbal medicines, unless prescribed by a physician over-seeing post-treatment care. Herbs contain a wealth of compounds, many of which have not yet been fully explored by scientists for their actions. Some of these plant chemicals are cytotoxic, meaning they indiscriminately kill cells. As such, it is strongly recommended that all such supplements be stopped for at least one month (the timeframe during which stem-cell migration, engraftment, and pro-liferation takes place).

- The effect of many vitamins and antioxidants on stem-cell activity is unknown. As such, it is best to err on the side of caution and stop using all such supplements (except for those specifically recom-mended in this book or by a physician in charge of post-hUCSC treatment care). This restriction is observed for at least one month following stem-cell therapy.

- No red meat or heat-processed, cholesterol-rich foods such as eggs, aged cheese, fried or baked foods, or dairy products for at least ninety days following treatment. These foods contain oxidized cholesterol (oxysterols) and other compounds that may interfere with cell-pro-liferation activities.

- Nuts and seeds are forbidden for the first two to three months following hUCSC treatment, especially in people with progressive neurological conditions such as MS and ALS. This food group is rich in the amino acid L-arginine, which is turned into the compound nitric oxide in the central nervous system. Nitric oxide is detrimental for people with many neurological and other challenges because it fuels neuroinflammation, much like throwing gas on a fire. Comparisons done by SRI staff of MS patients who received hUCSC therapy and ate nuts and seeds during the first sixty days following treatment, with those who did not indicates that the latter group did far, far better.

Factors That Tend to Increase Stem-Cell Growth

Patients enrolled in the Ramirez hUCSC therapy program are counseled to do the following during the first three days following a stem-cell injection.

- **Eat foods containing calcium, magnesium, potassium, and B complex, or that promote production of the mood-modulating neurotransmitter serotonin.** These nutrients help reduce stress and depression and thus may bring about hormonal and biochemical conditions in body tissues that tend to support and sustain cell proliferation. Among the foods recommended are:
  - **Serotonin-generating foods:** Squash, pumpkin, turnips, and celery. (Do not eat any brown spots on celery. They can promote free radical damage.)
  - **Calcium-rich foods:** Salmon, sardines, green leafy vegetables, collards, filberts, kale, kelp, mustard greens, prunes, turnip greens, and watercress.
  - **Magnesium-rich foods:** Avocados, brewer's yeast, dulse, green leafy vegetables, salmon, and watercress.
  - **Potassium-rich foods:** Avocados, brewer's yeast, dulse, raisins, and winter squash.
  - **B complex-rich foods:**
    - **Folic acid:** Green leafy vegetables, asparagus, and spinach.
    - **Pyridoxine (vitamin B_6) and methylcobalamin (a form of vitamin B_{12}):** Poultry, fish oil, vegetables.

- **Eat zinc-rich foods.** Zinc is important in protein synthesis and nerve development and maintenance. Foods rich in zinc include eggs, turkey, sunflower seeds, and sesame seeds.

- **Eat lots of fish and seafood high in the omega-3 fatty acid DHA (docosahexaenoic acid), while avoiding fish that contains high levels of mercury.** (See "Mercury in Fish" below for specifics.) The omega-3 fatty acids play a role in nerve-cell growth, cognition, and modulating inflammatory responses. Wild-caught salmon is especially rich in omega-3 rich fatty acids and is low in mercury. (Fish-farm salmon has been found to contain high levels of mercury and should be avoided.)

- **Supplement with ginseng.** The compounds in ginseng, known as

---

Mercury in Fish

Mercury is toxic to existing and new neurons. Therefore, it is important to eat only types of fish that contain low levels of this element.

High to Moderate Levels of Mercury

- *Crab, canned*
- *Halibut*
- *Lobster*
- *Mackerel*
- *Shark*
- *Swordfish*
- *Tilefish*
- *White tuna, canned*

Low Levels of Mercury

- *Clams*
- *Oysters*
- *Pollack*
- *Salmon*
- *Sardines*
- *Scallops*
- *Shrimp*
- *Tuna, light*

Source: American Heart Association, Food & Drug Administration.

ginsenosides, have been reported to increase stem-cell proliferation. The doctors doing hUCSC therapy generally recommend using Chinese ginseng or blends of ginsengs (Korean, Chinese) that are known to be rich in ginsenosides, for anywhere from three to six months or longer following hUCSC therapy.

CONCLUSION

The diet advocated by SRI and the research-oriented doctors doing hUCSC therapy in Mexico is geared to line up with what our ancestors ate and thrived on for millions of years prior to the advent of agriculture. It is relatively high in "good" fats and high-protein sources, such as certain cold-water species of fish and game meats, as well as lots of vegetables and certain fruits. Grains and cereals are not allowed because they generate compounds that tend to fuel neuroinflammation, bind needed minerals like calcium, and in many instances, supply gluten, which a great many people are sensitive to. Milk is eliminated because it contains casein and other substances that can exacerbate inflammatory processes in the central nervous system. Nuts and seeds are forbidden because they increase production of nitric oxide in the central nervous system, and nitric acid contributes to neuroinflammation.

Since 2003, patients on the SRI diet have generally had better healing responses to hUCSC treatment than those who did not follow it. This reaction has been especially true of adults and children with progressive neurological disorders that involve inflammation. On the other hand, infants and small children who do not have conditions based on or contributed to by neuroinflammation do fairly well, even without strictly adhering to the dietary protocols. Adults, especially older ones, benefit from the diet whether or not they have a progressive neurologic disorder or disease.

CHAPTER 7

Natural Methods of Stem-Cell Renewal

I n this chapter, we will look at scientifically validated ways in which anyone reading this book can help insure that the stem cells residing throughout their bodies are not compromised in terms of their function or ability to mobilize in response to injury or disease by dietary and other factors. Furthermore, ways and means to help get stem cells mobilized from one's bone marrow and into the circulatory system will also be discussed.

It is important to understand that evidence is increasingly coming to light that relates aging and disease to a lack of normal stem-cell growth and repair. If a person develops a degenerative disease, it is in part because the person's stem cells are either inhibited from growing or are destroyed at a faster rate than they can be produced. If stem cells are not being produced to help replace injured and worn-out tissue, the balance between growth and decline shifts toward decline. A more sweeping, integrative approach to health and healing is fast emerging that is aimed at determining which lifestyle practices, therapies, medications, and supplements are beneficial by how they affect the body's normal repair and regenerative processes. This exciting new clinical arena is endogenous stem-cell mobilization—the ability to mobilize a person's own stem cells for brain repair and regeneration.

THE NATURAL PRODUCTION OF
STEM CELLS IN ADULTS

Before discussing the factors that support and inhibit normal stem-cell growth, note that neural stem/progenitor cells *can* be produced in adults. Forty years ago, researchers observed that new neurons could be formed in the rat brain after birth.[1] This observation was contrary to the prevailing belief that neurons were the one cell in the body that could not be replaced—we could increase the connections (synapses) between neurons but not the neurons themselves. It took another thirty years to chisel away at the old beliefs and replace them with a view of the brain that includes life-long stem-cell renewal.

While new stem cells have been observed to develop in various areas of the brain, there seem to be two major regions that act like neural stem-cell nurseries. One area is called the "dentate gyrus," located in the hippocampus, a region of the brain devoted to learning and memory. In a second area, neural stem cells originate near the cerebellum (important for coordinated movement) and then travel to the olfactory bulb in the nose. If there is an injury in the brain, these neural stem cells travel to the damaged tissue rather than continuing along their path to the olfactory bulb. This is the reason why the lack of smell is now being used as a simple screening tool to help diagnose brain injury and Alzheimer's disease.[2, 3] If fewer stem cells are reaching the olfactory bulb, there will be less developing neurons to provide the sense of smell.

The knowledge that the brain produces stem cells that can help maintain its functioning and effect repairs when it is diseased or injured is most reassuring.

HOW WE CAN ASSIST THE PROCESS
OF CREATING NEW NEURONS AND
HOW WE CAN AVOID IMPEDING IT

There are a number of things that can hinder stem-cell activity or even kill them off, and do and not do to help promote greater health and longevity as individuals and as a society. The "not do's" are the factors that injure and kill neural stem cells, progenitor cells, and new neurons. (A stem cell can beget another stem cell or a neural stem cell. The neural stem cell can beget a neural progenitor, and the neural progenitor can beget a new neuron.) The "not do's" include the following: air, water, and land pollution; toxic pesticides and herbicides; metal and chemical toxicity; pathogens; radiation; drinking alcohol; smoking and using tobacco and tobacco products; use of cocaine and other illicit drugs; sleep deprivation and sleep apnea; excessive stress; allergies; inflammation; and a poor diet. All of these factors produce free radicals. Free radicals are unpaired electrons that break apart other molecules such as proteins and DNA. When more free radicals are generated than the body can handle, they will induce a cell (including a brain cell) to destroy itself. This self-destruct process is called "programmed cell death," or apoptosis. Enzymes are released that break apart protein bonds and divide up the cell into small pieces. Then immune cells called "phagocytes" come in and ingest the remains. Until free radicals are reduced in the body, there is also a risk of increased genetic instability that leads to the production of cancer cells rather than normal stem cells.

The following are factors that can promote the growth of normal stem cells. Much of this information has already been presented in this book because nurturing stem cells after stem-cell therapy is similar to nurturing the growth, proliferation, and differentiation of our own endogenous (produced in the body) stem cells. In fact, we are learning that many of the factors presented in health and longevity books promote health and longevity because they support normal stem-cell renewal.

1. Detoxification

Removing impediments that might hinder the body from creating normal stem cells is a logical, sensible measure, which is often called "detoxification" by many physicians. This process includes checking for and correcting gut dysbiosis ("leaky gut"), heavy metal toxicity, infections, and inflammation.

2. Promoting Balance between the Sympathetic and Parasympathetic Nervous System

In high-school health classes, many of us learned about the sympathetic nervous system (the flight-or-fight stress response) and the parasympathetic nervous system (for maintenance and repair). The stress response releases hormones, such as cortisol, from the adrenal glands that reduce pain and inflammation. However, these hormones also stimulate an excitatory neurotransmitter called "glutamate." In small amounts, glutamate stimulates the growth of neural stem cells and plays an important role in learning and memory. However, in higher concentrations, as with acute and chronic stress, glutamate is toxic to neural progenitor cells and new neurons. The chronic loss of neurons over the years from stress-induced glutamate toxicity is considered a risk factor for memory loss and Alzheimer's disease.[4]

Because modern life is so fast paced, much of the workday for many people can be characterized as sympathetic nervous system activation. However, this also inhibits the parasympathetic functions of repair, which appears to negatively impact the proliferation of new stem/progenitor cells for regeneration.[5] To allow for greater balance and greater health, some moments in each day should be dedicated to physiological and psychological peace. This can mean watching a sunrise or sunset, reading inspirational or humorous books and articles, a creative project, prayer, meditation, deep breathing, massage, enjoying the company of others, and so on.

An activity that is relaxing (that is, reduces heart rate and blood pressure[6]) also increases serotonin in the brain and serotonin regulates neural stem-cell growth.[7] Elevated levels of serotonin increase the production of new neurons in the dentate gyrus (in the hippocampus) and serotonin deficiency or inhibition decreases the number of new neurons. Serotonin plays a role in estrogen's ability to stimulate neural cell growth in the dentate gyrus.[8] Antidepressants that increase serotonin levels in the brain also promote neural stem-cell growth.

Certain foods, such as turkey, contain the amino acid tryptophan, which increases brain serotonin levels. In addition, serotonin is required for the production of melatonin, an anti-aging hormone of the pineal gland. Foods that tend to favor serotonin/melatonin synthesis in the body include squash, pumpkin, carrots, onions, garlic, turnips, celery, cabbage, cauliflower, tomatoes, cucumber, radishes, pomegranate, strawberry, and ginger. By consuming these foods at dinnertime, we can help promote relaxation, as well as repair and regeneration once we fall asleep.

3. Sleep Is a Restorative Process That Includes Stem-Cell Proliferation

The "sleep-promoting hormone" melatonin is beneficial in several ways: It helps to regulate the circadian rhythms (twenty-four-hour cycle), core body temperature, immune function, and sleep-wake cycles. Melatonin is also a powerful antioxidant that protects against free-radical damage. In addition, normal physiologic levels of melatonin are associated with increasing neural stem-cell proliferation in the hippocampus.[9] In fact, the process of sleep itself may be an orchestration of growth factors and electrical activity that promotes stem-cell growth, proliferation, and differentiation.

On the flip side, sleep deprivation reduces stem-cell proliferation.[10] For example, rats deprived of sleep for forty-eight hours showed a dramatic reduction in neural stem cells in the hippocampus, and this reduction required more than eight hours of recovery sleep to reverse. Also, melatonin levels decrease and sleep quality declines with age. In fact, some doctors actually link some key aspects of aging to a melatonin deficiency.[11] Generally speaking, thirty-five-year-olds have an average nighttime melatonin level of 90 picograms(pg)/milliliter (mL) whereas seventy-year-olds have an average of 30 pg/mL, which is a significant difference. For this reason, many physicians now recommend that older people bring their melatonin level up to a more youthful level.

Melatonin supplements taken at night have been used by people of all ages to reduce disorders associated with sleep disturbance. Melatonin supplementation has also been reported to improve function in stroke, Alzheimer's disease, Parkinson's disease, Huntington's disease, radiation, diabetes, viral infections, glutamate toxicity, metal toxicity, and seizures.[12]

Growth hormone (GH) is also released during sleep. Growth-hormone deficiency is associated with impaired cognitive and cardiovascular function in aging rats,[13] whereas GH treatment partially improves these functions.[14] In addition, the number of neurons was reduced in the hippocampus of aging rats, and GH treatment significantly increased new neurons. GH deficiency from pituitary dysfunction is often seen in traumatic brain injury and should be considered in a treatment program.[15]

For several years, it became popular to take the amino acid supplement arginine to increase the body's growth hormone, but this is not advisable. Although flooding the body with high-dose L-arginine orally or by intravenous drip (IV) encourages the body to produce GH, it also helps produce nitric oxide, which can be a friend or foe. In the cardiovascular system, nitric oxide relaxes and dilates the blood vessels. This can help reduce heart rate and blood pressure. In the a normal, healthy person's hippocampus, nitric oxide helps set the stage for production of new neurons.[16] However, in the injured and aging brain, nitric oxide can also escalate inflammation and free-radical damage. Together with hydrogen peroxide, nitric oxide can form peroxynitrite, which is highly toxic to neurons. An alternative to L-arginine for promoting GH may be the combination of aged garlic extract and a powerful antioxidant compound from conifer tree bark (like pine) called Pycnogenol.[17] Soy lecithin contains GPC (glycerylphosphorylcholine), which also promotes growth hormone production.[18]

A different approach to increasing growth hormone is to maintain sufficient levels of calcium in the diet (with a 1:1 or 2:1 ratio with magnesium). Calcium deficiency stimulates the production of parathyroid hormone. Even slight elevations of parathyroid hormone can reduce growth hormone levels by 50 percent.[19] This being the case, undergoing tests to determine if one's calcium level is normal and, if not, taking calcium supplements with follow-up testing and dosage adjustments would be prudent.

Although no one can say with absolute certainty why we sleep, one benefit of it appears to be the release of hormones such as melatonin and growth factor, along with a host of other factors that help maintain health and possibly encourage stem-cell proliferation and activity.

4. Vitamin D Promotes the Growth of New Neurons

Sunlight is a major source of vitamin D, and throughout history, light has been associated with intelligence and wisdom. Is this association just symbolic? There have been stories about people being kept in dark dungeons in medieval times so they would be mindless followers. Part of the reason for their diminished mental powers as well as a short and weakened skeletal structure may be a lack of sunlight and vitamin D. Vitamin D helps regulate calcium levels, bone mineralization, immune function, and cell differentiation. It also stimulates growth factors for brain development. Vitamin D_3 can promote nerve growth factor, glial cell-derived neurotrophic factor, and brain-derived neurotrophic factor.[20,21] These growth factors are important in promoting stem-cell growth, proliferation, and differentiation into brain cells—neurons, glia, and astrocytes (neurons are called "gray matter"; and glia and astrocytes are "white matter cells" that nourish and protect the neurons). Morning sunlight and full-spectrum indoor light have been effective in reducing the symptoms of sleep deprivation, sleep disorders, and depression.[22,23] Light therapy may benefit by inducing new stem-cell growth and by resetting the circadian clock. Vitamin D_3 can reduce the amount of brain damage caused by stroke in laboratory animals.[24] It also protects dopamine neurons from toxicity in patients with Parkinson's disease.[25] Dietary sources of vitamin D include fish oil, dairy products (watch for allergies), and vitamin D supplements (in moderation).

5. Lifelong Learning Increases the Production of New Stem Cells

Going back to our medieval imprisonment example, keeping someone "in the dark" can also refer to a lack of information and mental stimulation. The hippocampus is important for learning and memory. Thousands of new stem/progenitor cells are produced each day in a part of the hippocampus called the "dentate gyrus." Learning helps these cells survive and vice versa; the development of these cells helps improve learning and memory.

An enriched, complex environment for rats that fosters new opportunities for learning and social interaction increases the growth of new neurons in the dentate gyrus and promotes improved long-term memory.[26] New neurons in the dentate gyrus have calcium and sodium action potentials that are different from those of older neurons. These action potentials make new neurons better able to achieve "long-term potentiation," a physiological function associated with creating new memories.[27] In addition, an enriched environment was found to reduce beta-amyloid levels and deposits in laboratory animals. Beta-amyloid peptides are toxic to neurons in the hippocampus. These peptides are associated with neuronal loss and cognitive decline in Alzheimer's disease.

Learning not only reduces the formation of beta-amyloid peptides, but it can also increase new blood vessels (for increased oxygen) and neuroprotective factors for greater brain-cell survival.[28] Learning after a stroke in laboratory animals has also been found to help stimulate stem-cell repair and reduce the amount of brain damage caused by the stroke.[29]

From this body of laboratory research, we are discovering that those who continue to learn new things throughout their lives and see things from a new perspective may also be stimulating the growth factors in the brain to produce new stem cells and new neurons. These new neurons provide an improved ability to create and recall new memories. In addition, these growth factors may also help improve function in neurological injuries and disorders.

6. The Impact of Stress on Endogenous Stem-Cell Activity and New Neuron Formation

Have you ever memorized a speech and literally knew it backward and forward only to forget it when you had to recite it in front of other people? If so, you know firsthand that stress can interfere with learning and memory. It can also lead to learning disabilities and feelings of defeat. Stress-induced corticosterone (and glucocosteroid-induced glutamate) in the dentate gyrus injure neural stem/progenitor cells and reduce our capacity to learn and remember recent events. In addition, stress in childhood can remain as neural deficits in the adult. In animal studies, rat pups that experienced maternal deprivation showed heightened and prolonged corticosterone release to mild stresses as adults. The outcome was chronic stress-induced neuronal injury and death so that as adults, the rats showed significantly reduced neurons in the hippocampus.[30] Similar findings for reduced neurons in the hippocampus have resulted from prenatal stress in rhesus monkeys.[31] There are also studies that show differences in stem/progenitor cell activity and dominant and submissive character traits. Aged, dominant mice were found to have more brain-derived neurotrophic factor that promotes neural stem-cell proliferation, whereas aged, submissive mice had increased levels of nerve growth factor. Nerve growth factor can be increased by stress, including emotional stresses of fear and anxiety, to help protect against neural cell death in the hippocampus.[32] These research studies suggest that stress in pregnancy and during childhood can lead to reduced brain development and a reduced capacity for learning and memory in the hippocampus. In addition, chronic stress can lead to psychological submission, defeat, and depression, characterized by reduced stem-cell renewal in the dentate gyrus of the hippocampus.

The negative effects of stress on the body can be reduced by taking neuroprotective antioxidants such as N-acetyl-cysteine (which increases glutathione production); R-lipoic acid; melatonin; the omega-3 fatty acid DHA (in fish oil): ginseng; *Ginkgo biloba*; vitamins B_6, C, D, and E; beta-carotene (those who smoke or who once did should consult a physician about the use of beta-carotene, since it caused an increase in lung cancer during one major clinical trial); curcumin in turmeric root (used in curry powder blends); Pycnogenol (pine bark); garlic; taurine; green tea and green tea extract; and resveratrol (in grape juice and red wine; however, those with brain injuries should avoid alcohol, including red wine). Naturally when to take these supplements and how much must be worked out with a physician or dietician who is knowledgeable concerning the best forms, potential drug interactions, and how to monitor bodily response.

7. Supporting Mitochondrial Function

The mitochondria are little energy factories in the cell that produce a compound called "adenosine triphosphate" (ATP) that basically powers cellular activities. If ATP levels diminish, free-radical levels increase, often causing cell death. Mitochondrial support through optimal nutrition is important to reduce free-radical damage and DNA instability. In addition to antioxidants, factors that support mitochondrial function include coenzyme Q_{10} and Idebenone (a form of coenzyme Q_{10}), acetyl-L-carnitine, R- and alpha-lipoic acid, and a form of niacin called nicotinamide. Nutrients that support DNA stability and repair include niacin, folic acid, vitamin B_{12} (as methylcobalamin rather than cyanocobalamin), vitamin C (helps to stabilize the extracellular matrix), and vitamin D (helps to stabilize the chromosome structure). DNA and mitochondrial support are very important, especially in times of stress, for promoting the growth of normal stem cells.

8. Moderate Exercise Is a Leading Factor in Promoting Longevity

Exercise promotes the growth of new stem cells. Although extreme exercise increases free-radical damage, moderate exercise is a health-promoting activity. Moderate exercise increases VEGF (vascular endothelial growth factor) to stimulate the growth of new blood vessels. This supplies increased oxygen and nutrients to the cells (including brain cells). Exercise—especially complex movements such as gymnastics—promotes brain integration and stimulates the release of BDNF (brain-derived neurotrophic factor). BDNF promotes the growth of new stem/progenitor cells in the hippocampus. It also promotes the switching on (upregulation) of genes that increase neural plasticity, including the growth of synapses that connect one neuron to another. Exercise is also an antidote for stress, depression, and anxiety.[33] Much has been written about the health-promoting benefits of caloric restriction. Caloric restriction also increases BDNF and stem-cell renewal.[34] However, for those who are not apt to reduce their food intake, exercise offers similar benefits.

9. Mobilizing Bone-Marrow Stem Cells Promotes Stem-Cell Renewal

Brown seaweed contains compounds called "fucoidans" that have a number of interesting benefits. Certain forms of them that readily get into the body can reduce blood coagulation like the blood-thinning drug heparin but without the risk of internal bleeding.[35] Fucoidans can bind with fibroblast growth factors which can then stimulate the development of new blood vessels (angiogenesis) in damaged tissue. At the same time, fucoidans also inhibit the growth of smooth muscle cells. A characteristic of atherosclerosis is the proliferation of smooth muscle cells inside the blood vessel walls so that they gradually block the flow of blood through the arteries and blood vessels. Fucoidans appear to help to favorably impact this atherosclerotic process, perhaps by anti-inflammatory and stem-cell repair processes. Fucoidans also induce rapid bone marrow stem-cell mobilization into the bloodstream.[36] This mobilization of bone-marrow stem/progenitor cells can help repair injuries throughout the cardiovascular system as well as promote renewal in the brain.[37,38] The challenge is reducing inflammation and free-radical production so that the progenitor cells are not injured and destroyed.

CONCLUSION

We all enter this world with a unique complement of defenses and restorative mechanisms to help us survive and surmount the "trails and tribulations" that life throws at us. Our bodies maintain a vigilant surveillance for threats to health and well-being, and work diligently to maintain balance (homeostasis) and stave off disease and facilitate repair and replacement of diseased or defective cells and tissues. This innate biologic arsenal includes stem cells that reside in tissues and organs throughout our bodies, which serve to create new cells lost to disease, age, or injury. But it is a "defense and repair force" that requires support in the form of sound nutrition, sleeping patterns, and adoption of health-conducive lifestyle measures. There are also measures that can be taken that may help mobilize one's own stem cells from the bone marrow and by so doing make them available for "maintenance and repair duty." Among those discussed in this chapter are reduction of stress and inflammation, staying physically and mentally active, along with the medically informed and appropriate use of such "brain, body, and endogenous stem-cell friendly" compounds as N-acetyl-cysteine, acetyl-L-carnitine, R-lipoic acid, melatonin, the omega-3 fatty acid DHA (in fish oil), ginseng, *Ginkgo biloba* extract, vitamins B$_6$, C, D, and full-spectrum vitamin E, curcumin extract (plus curry powder in foods), Pycnogenol (pine bark), garlic, L-taurine, green tea and green tea extract, certain fucoidan-rich brown seaweed formulations, and resveratrol.

The Road to Improvement for Many

A woman who was paralyzed for nineteen years was able to stand and move her legs following a hUCSC implant performed by scientists at South Korea's Chosun University. More than twenty children with cerebral palsy and more than ten with traumatic brain injury treated with hUCSCs since 2003 have shown marked improvements that include cases of reduced spasticity, the resolution of cortical blindness and aphasia (inability to speak), and an increased ability to move around. Three children who were cortically blind began tracking objects with their eyes within three months of receiving a single hUCSC treatment. A four-year-old girl with a terminal genetic neurological disorder that isn't supposed to improve went from being cortically blind and having a limp to being able to move her limbs and track objects with her eyes within two months of receiving 1.5 million CD34+/CD45(–) hUCSCs.

In some ways, it would seem that science has caught up with biblical accounts of the blind seeing and the lame walking. And, to a degree, it has, as is amply illustrated in the patient accounts contained in this book. However, it would be presumptive to characterize hUCSC therapy as affording suffering individuals anything approaching a miraculous medical turnaround. Yet even so, the artful application of hUCSC therapy appears to produce medically significant benefits in many non-hematopoietic (non-blood-related) diseases and conditions.

Critics, of course, point out that many of the people who have shown improvements following hUCSC therapy would have done so anyway due to the nature of their condition, which is to say, some diseases or medical issues get better as the body grows or otherwise changes with the passage of time or as the results wrought by other therapies kick in. This certainly may be true in some cases. However, the type, degree, and swiftness of improvements that have followed on the heels of hUCSC therapy in many cases suggest that the stem cells themselves are helping bring about healing or restoration.

If one grants, however tentatively, that umbilical-cord stem-cell therapy does bring about beneficial changes in either sick or physically or mentally challenged people, how does it do so? Are the stem cells traveling to the brains of children with cerebral palsy or traumatic brain injury and transforming into neurons, thereby accounting for the improvements that follow? Some experts say this is unlikely unless the cells are placed directly into the brain. However, animal studies show that hUCSCs injected in the tail vein migrate through the blood-brain barrier. When hUCSCs are introduced into rats with induced strokes via their tail vein, the stem cells have been shown to penetrate the blood-brain barrier, make their way into the animal's brains, and initiate a healing response. Examination of the rat's brains has revealed the presence of the human umbilical-cord stem cells integrated into the brain tissue, bearing neural markers (a biochemical signature common to specific types of neurons).

But is this happening in the children who receive this therapy as well? They are receiving subcutaneous injections of between 1.5–2.8 million hUCSCs into tissue near their belly buttons, although some have received IV infusions of hUCSCs. Are these hUCSCs somehow finding their way into the children's circulations and then migrating into their brains and becoming new neurons? We simply don't know. It may well be that any cells that do make it into the brain are acting as "nurse cells" or "chaperones," meaning that they are coaxing damaged cells to function better by producing specific growth factors or other compounds or cofactors that foster healing, regeneration, or repair. Or it may be that the hUCSC injected into subcutaneous fatty tissue is causing fat cells to churn out compounds such as tumor necrosis factor-alpha (TNF-a), which opens up the blood-brain barrier, and other compounds such as nerve growth factor (NGF), which facilitates the creation of new neurons or the healing of damaged ones.

As this book goes to press, Steenblock Research Institute's in-house laboratory is collecting pre- and post-hUCSC therapy blood samples from patients and doing tests to measure levels of TNF-a and NGF. The results may reveal one way in which hUCSCs could be working to bring about the type and kind of medical improvements seen in patients treated in Mexico and elsewhere.

The absence of a demonstrated mechanism for how hUCSCs can affect neurological repair is not, however, sufficient cause to write off their use—especially for intractable conditions and those for which the best available therapies can afford only modest gains. In the history of medicine, many drugs have been employed—sometimes for decades—without our knowing exactly how they worked. Many only produced benefit in a subset of the patients treated. The real issues, then, boil down to safety and effectiveness.

When it comes to the use of matched cord blood and unmatched pure hUCSCs, the track record with respect to safety appears very solid. And while their effectiveness for various non-hematopoietic (especially neurological) disorders and diseases is not proved in controlled studies yet, a sufficient body of case history data and preliminary results from small studies exist to suggest that hUCSC therapy is producing genuine repair and healing. For many people and doctors too, these results are sufficient to venture into what is surely only a partially explored frontier.

So, why should, say, acute stroke patients or parents of children with crippling cerebral palsy or traumatic brain injury not wait for the results of formal controlled studies before trying an admittedly experimental treatment like hUCSC therapy? In a word, what compels most to press on is their individual biological window of opportunity. Stroke damage heals over and with this healing, it would seem, the chemical signals that attract stem cells to the site of injury diminish. Aging itself brings about bodily changes that appear to blunt responses to hUCSC therapy, which suggests that "younger is better" in terms of being treated (at least this is the pattern that has emerged in the 100-plus cases accrued and analyzed at Steenblock Research Institute). And since no one, it would seem, gets worse as a result of the treatment (no harm is done short or long term), it seems more ethical in the minds of many to do the treatment than to forgo it.

Bottom line: hUCSCs do not work miracles by any stretch of the imagination. Published studies do point to their being safe and effective for many hematopoietic diseases and disorders. And now evidence is accruing that suggests these cells can bring about improvements in adults and children with various neurological, eye, and circulatory diseases and conditions.

It is often necessary to take a decision on the basis of knowledge sufficient for action, but insufficient to satisfy the intellect.

—IMMANUEL KANT

Glossary

Adult stem cell—An undifferentiated cell found in a differentiated tissue that can renew itself and differentiate (with certain limitations) to produce all the specialized cell types of the tissue from which it originated.

Astrocyte—One of the large glia cells found in neural tissues.

Blastocyst—A preimplantation embryo consisting of about 150 cells. The blastocyst consists of a sphere made up of an outer layer of cells (the trophoectoderm), a fluid-filled cavity (the blastocoel), and a cluster of cells on the interior (the inner cell mass).

Bone-marrow stromal cells—A stem cell found in bone marrow that generates bone, cartilage, fat, and fibrous connective tissue.

CD34+ stem cells—A very primitive human umbilical-cord stem cell.

Cell culture—Growth of cells in a petri dish or other vessel (referred to as "in vitro") on an artificial medium for experimental research.

Cell division—Method by which a single cell divides to create two cells. This continuous process allows a population of cells to increase or maintain its numbers.

Cell-based therapies—Treatment in which stem cells are induced to differentiate into the specific cell type required to repair injured, diseased, infected, or depleted adult-cell populations or tissues.

Chelation therapy—Oral or IV therapy that helps remove toxic heavy metals like lead, mercury, and iron from a patient's body.

Clone—A line of cells that is genetically identical to the originating cell.

Cloning—The transplantation of a nucleus from a nonegg, nonsperm, nonstem cell into a egg, which then develops into an embryo.

Culture medium—A broth that sustains cells in a culture or petri dish. It often contains nutrients to feed the cells as well as other growth factors that may be added to direct desired changes in the cells.

Cytokines—Small but highly potent proteins that modulate the activity of many cell types.

Differentiation—Refers to a process whereby an unspecialized early embryonic cell acquires the features of a specialized cell such as a heart, liver, or muscle cell.

DNA—Deoxyribonucleic acid, a chemical found primarily in the nucleus of cells. DNA carries the blueprint for making all the structures and materials the body needs to function.

D.O.—Doctor of Osteopathy—D.O.s are fully qualified physicians who can dispense drugs, do surgery, and deliver babies. They are licensed in all fifty states.

Ectoderm—Upper, outermost layer of a group of cells derived from the inner cell mass of the blastocyst, which gives rise to skin and brain nerves.

Embryo—The term embryo refers to an animal or a plant in its earliest stage of development; in humans, the term refers to the developing organism from the time of fertilization until the end of the eighth week of gestation.

Embryonic stem cells—Primitive (undifferentiated) cells found in embryos that have the potential to become a wide variety of specialized cell types.

Embryonic stem-cell line—Embryonic stem cells, which have been cultured in the laboratory (in vitro) so as to allow proliferation without differentiation for months or longer.

Endoderm—Lower layer of a group of cells derived from the inner cell mass of the blastocyst, which gives rise to lungs and digestive organs.

Feeder layer—Cells used as part of cultures that maintain pluripotent stem cells in the laboratory. These feeder cells often consist of mouse embryonic fibroblasts.

Fertilization—The process whereby male sperm and the female egg (ovum) unite.

Fetus—Refers to a developing human from about two months after conception to birth.

Gene—Refers to a segment of DNA located in a specific site on a chromosome. (Humans have 46 chromosomes in each cell of their bodies.) Genes are the basic unity of heredity in that they direct the formation of enzymes or other proteins.

Glaucoma—An eye disease in which the normal fluid pressure inside the eyes slowly rises, leading to vision loss or blindness.

Growth factors—Compounds produced by the body that control growth, division, and maturation of cells and tissues.

Hematopoietic stem cell—Stem cell from which all red and white blood cells develop, and which can also generate certain immune cells. Laboratory studies indicate that these stem cells can become cells with characteristics of neurons, liver cells, heart cells, and as well as other cells.

Host versus graft reaction—Immune system rejection of a transplanted organ or tissue or cells.

Human embryonic stem cell—A type of pluripotent stem cell found in the inner cell mass of the blastocyst.

Hypoxia—A deficiency of oxygen in a tissue or tissues or organ or organs in the body.

In vitro—A Latin term that means "in glass," as in a laboratory dish or test tube; an artificial environment.

Inner cell mass—A cluster of cells inside the blastocyst, which give rise to the embryonic disk of the later embryo and, ultimately, the fetus.

Long-term self-renewal—The ability of stem cells to renew themselves by dividing into the same nonspecialized cell type over long periods of time (from months to years) depending on the specific type of stem cell.

Macular degenerative—A chronic disease of the eyes caused by the deterioration of the central portion of the retina, known as the macula, which is critical for focusing central vision.

Matrix metalloproteinases—Enzymes that use a metal such as zinc and degrade the extracellular matrix (the microenvironment around cells that supports and influences them). They play an important role in several neurodegenerative processes.

Mesenchymal stem cells—Cells found in the immature embryonic connective tissue or from the umbilical cord. A number of cell types are generated by mesenchymal stem cells, including chondrocytes, which produce cartilage.

Mesoderm—Middle layer of a group of cells derived from the inner cell mass of the blastocyst, which gives rise to bone, muscle, and connective tissue.

Microenvironment—Refers to the molecules, compounds, and cells including nutrients and growth factors in the fluid or matrix surrounding a cell in an organism or in the laboratory. The microenvironment plays an important role in determining the characteristics of a cell.

Multiple sclerosis—A chronic degenerative disease of the central nervous system in which the insulation around nerves called "myelin" is eroded or missing in patches called lesions throughout the brain or spinal cord (or both), interfering with the nerve function and causing muscular weakness, loss of coordination and speech, and visual disturbances. (In healthy people myelin is not eroded or missing.)

Multipotent stem cells—Refers to stem cells that can give rise to several other cell types, but those types are limited in number.

Neural stem cell—A stem cell found in adult brain and nerve tissue that can give rise to neurons, astrocytes, and oligodendrocytes.

Neurons—Refers to nerve cells, the structural and functional unit of the nervous system, which consist of a cell body and its processes, an axon, and one or more dendrites. Neurons function by initiating and conducting impulses and transmitting impulses to other neurons or cells by releasing neurotransmitters at synapses.

Oligodendrocyte—A cell that provides insulation to nerve cells by forming a myelin sheath around axons, similar to insulation around a wire in an electrical appliance or home.

Placenta—An organ rich in blood vessels that develops in female mammals during pregnancy, and which lines the uterine wall and partially envelopes the fetus. The fetus is attached to the placenta by the umbilical cord. The placenta is expelled from the mother's body following birth.

Plasticity—The ability of stem cells from one adult tissue to generate differentiated cell types of another kind of tissue.

Pluripotent—Refers to the ability of a single stem cell to develop into many different cell types of the body.

Pluripotent stem cells—Pluripotent refers to stem cells that are able to differentiate into many cell types. Pluripotent stem cells can eventually specialize in any bodily tissue, but they cannot themselves develop into a human being.

Proliferation—Refers to expansion of a population of cells by continuous division.

Regenerative or reparative medicine—Refers to medical therapy or treatment in which stem cells are induced to differentiate into the specific cell types required to repair damaged, traumatized, infected, or depleted adult-cell populations or tissues.

Signals—Internal and external biochemical factors that control changes in cell structure and function.

Somatic stem cells—Another name for adult stem cells.

Stem cells—Refers to cells with the ability to divide for indefinite periods in culture and to give rise to specialized cells.

Stromal cells—Non-blood cells derived from blood-producing organs, such as bone marrow or fetal liver. These cells are capable of supporting growth of blood cells in vitro. Stromal cells that make up the matrix within the bone marrow are also derived from mesenchymal stem cells.

Surface markers—Cell surface proteins that are unique to certain cell types. They can be visualized using antibodies that attach to them or by other detection methods.

Teratoma—Refers to a tumor composed of tissues from the three embryonic germ layers, and usually found in the ovaries and testes. Teratomas have been produced experimentally in animals by injecting pluripotent embryonic stem cells.

Tissue inhibitors of metalloproteinases (TIMPs)—Groups of related proteins (TIMP-1, TIMP-2, and TIMP-3) secreted by cells or tissues that play a crucial role in regulating the activity of enzymes called metalloproteinases. (Metalloproteinases are secreted by hUCSCs and make it possible for them to migrate through the human body and engraft.)

Totipotent—Totipotency refers to the ability of a single cell, usually a stem cell, to divide and produce all the different kinds (differentiated cells) in an organism, including extraembryonic tissues.

Transdifferentiation—Refers to a property of stem cells in which those from one tissue may be able to differentiate into cells of another tissue.

Umbilical-cord blood-derived stem cells—Stem cells that are contained in cord blood and in the tissue of the cord itself.

Undifferentiated—Refers to cells that have not changed into a specialized cell type.

Ethics and Politics
of Stem-Cell Therapy

Many nations throughout the world are grappling with the direction stem-cell research will take. The most contentious area concerns embryonic stem cells, as these come from embryos whose use many people equate with taking a life or exploiting potential human life. The use of stem cells derived from umbilical-cord blood, bone marrow, or adult tissues is not opposed by most people, including clerics, scientists, religious laypeople, or atheists or agnostics. Among mainstream conservative religious bodies such as the Roman Catholic Church, and most Baptist and Orthodox Jewish organizations, there is little or no opposition to the use of cord-blood stem cells or stem cells derived from adult tissue such as bone and fat.

In August 2001, President Bush set policy by stating that federal funds could be used to do embryonic stem-cell research, but restricted such funding to embryonic stem cells taken from various embryos (referred to as stem-cell lines) in existence at that time. In this way, Bush ensured that federal monies would not be used for research involving new lines that would come about as a result of culling stem cells from embryos. (The embryos would then be destroyed.) This action did not make it illegal to create new stem-cell lines; it just forbade the awarding of federal taxpayer money to fund research involving these new lines. Laboratories and research centers that are privately funded are at liberty to work with any of the hundreds of embryonic stem-cell lines created after August 2001.

Jeffrey Drazen, editor of *the New England Journal of Medicine*, responded to this policy of restricting development of new embryonic stem-cell lines eligible for federal funding for research purposes by warning that "the best and the brightest will be going out of the country to do [stem-cell research]. We would hope that people will understand that you can't legislate away scientific progress." No doubt many, many people including scientists would say, "Oh, yes you can!" Governmental bodies can, in short, pass laws that make it difficult if not impossible to pursue research that could prove to be a gold mine of medical benefits.

Some countries, like Germany, have prohibited some types of stem-cell research altogether, such as cloning because of public concerns and also because of problems connected with cloned animals such as Dolly in England. Still others like Singapore, South Korea, China, and the United Kingdom are pouring money into stem-cell research and allowing scientists greater freedom, both in terms of access to various kinds of stem cells (especially embryonic) and in terms of the direction their research takes (such as which diseases or applications they want to pursue and the ways in which they will tackle using stem cells such as tissue engineering outside the body for eventual transplant use, creation of insulin-producing cells for implantation into the pancreas of diabetes, and so on). None, however, appears to be throwing ethics to the wind and allowing scientists to work without guidelines or oversight. In Singapore and many other countries, projects and experiments are reviewed and critiqued by bioethicists who are fully acquainted with the standards held up by such organizations as the United Nations and major scientific organizations such as the American Association for the Advancement of Science (AAAS).

While America still leads the world in terms of available embryonic stem-cell lines and publishes a wealth of studies concerning not only embryonic stem cells, but adult and umbilical cord as well, there is a very real possibility that the lead will be lost to countries in Asia or elsewhere. A survey of recent developments in many of the nations who are spearheading stem-cell work richly illustrates this point:

- In Korea in May 2005, Dr. Woo Suk Hwang and his colleagues at Seoul National University announced that they had cloned human embryos and extracted stem cells from them.

- In July 2005, the Histostem Corporation in Seoul, South Korea, announced they will build a 100-bed hospital on the southern resort island of Jeju that will be devoted to offering human umbilical-cord stem-cell treatments.

- The government of Singapore has committed $1.5 billion dollars to high-tech work including stem cells. Much of this work is going on within a mini-city devoted to research dubbed "Biopolis." Many American scientists can now be found among the ranks of those doing stem-cell research in Singapore.

- Israeli scientists are using embryonic stem cells as tools to address such longstanding human afflictions as diabetes, heart disease, and various forms of cancer. In 2004, the Israeli government invested $20 million to bring together hospital, academic centers, and private companies for the express purpose of doing leading-edge research, stem cell included.

- The Chinese government has lent its support and money to spearhead stem-cell research, as well as to forge partnerships with private industry. The Chinese have a less restrictive regulatory environment than that of most of the Western nations, an encouragement to many of their scientists to press the research envelope.

- The United Kingdom has been a trailblazer in many areas that touch upon the use of embryos, and developed technology in the 1970s that made "test-tube babies" possible as well as the cloning of various mammals, including that of the famed sheep "Dolly" in the late 1990s. In 2004, Britain became the first nation in the world to set up a national stem-cell bank.

America, however, may be poised to shoot ahead in the years to come. During November 2004, voters in California approved Proposition 71, which will make available $3 billion for state-sanctioned stem-cell research over a ten-year period. The state of California then created the Institute for Regenerative Medicine for the purpose of helping funnel this money into stem-cell research projects and experiments at various schools, institutes, medical centers, and labs across the state. This will include projects involving human umbilical-cord stem cells. Not surprisingly, lawsuits have been filed to challenge this move and try to halt the stem-cell research momentum in California. Their outcome will determine whether California can go on to fund work that stands a good chance of propelling America ahead of the competition on the stem-cell arena.

Also, a bill titled "Cord Blood Stem Cell Act of 2005" was introduced in Congress to establish a national cord blood bank that would make cord blood available for research and medical use purposes. In May 2005, the renamed bill now called "Stem Cell Therapeutic & Research Act of 2005" passed in the House by a vote of 431 to 1. The Senate's vote on this bill has been held up because of issues created by unrelated bills dealing with embryonic stem cells.

Battlefield Traumatic Brain Injury:

The Promise of Human Umbilical-Cord Stem Cells (An Open Proposal)

This essay was originally written in the form of a letter by coauthors Steenblock and Payne and submitted to the editors of the *New England Journal of Medicine*. It was not selected for publication, but was deemed of merit by many healthcare and science professionals who were subsequently privy to its content. A copy of this letter did make its way into the hands of U.S. Senator Sam Brownback (R-Kansas) who, SRI was told, is considering introducing legislation to include hUCSCs among the medical modalities to be made available to doctors tending brain-injured soldiers in Iraq.

The May 19, 2005, issue of the *New England Journal of Medicine* (NEJM) contained a compelling article on traumatic brain injuries among soldiers in Iraq (Perspective—"Traumatic Brain Injury in the War Zone" by Susan Okie, M.D.; Vol. 352:2043–2047) that appeared alongside a powerful editorial op-ed piece by Jeffrey M. Drazen, M.D., titled "Using Every Resource to Care for Our Casualties" (NEJM Vol. 352:2121). These articles succinctly captured the bittersweet side of medicine as it applies to soldiers who have received head wounds in the field: While battlefield gear and contemporary battlefield medical intervention saves the lives of soldiers who would no doubt have perished in earlier wars, it leaves many of them to wrestle with physical and mental challenges that bioscience and technology seems poised to address. Indeed, modern science possesses the wherewithal to effect repair and recovery in ways that were the stuff of science fiction only a decade or two ago. Dr. Drazen mentions a few of these marvels in process such as "biohybrid devices and neural prostheses such as artificial retinas." Naturally, many of these must await refinements and then go on to garner proof of safety and efficacy in properly designed and executed clinical studies.

One area of therapeutic promise mentioned by Dr. Drazen concerns embryonic stem cells to help facilitate neurologic repair in soldiers who've sustained traumatic brain injuries on the battlefield. Drazen laments the lack of uniformity in the guidelines governing embryonic stem-cell research nationwide and voices a heartfelt desire that we should "give our researchers the fiscal and research resources they need to potentially help wounded veterans return to full function."

The need for continued research with respect to embryonic stem cells is something most of us in the scientific community appear to support. The real question is one of utility: Embryonic stem cells are inherently unstable once removed from their native tissue niche and tend to form tumors (teratomas) in lab animals. Probably a decade or more of concerted research lies ahead before these cells can be administered to human patients. Given the many struggles going on at all levels with respect to getting this body of research into high gear, it would seem that the prospect of near-term use is a distant hope at best.

Is there a safe alternative to embryonic stem cells for ameliorating neurologic challenges such as battlefield TBIs? We feel there is: Umbilical-cord stem cells. Since early 2003 our institute has accrued case history documentation and data indicating that human umbilical-cord stem cells can and do produce clinically significant responses in many common neurologic diseases and disorders. During 2004 our institute played an integral role in a pilot study involving eight children with cerebral palsy who were treated with a single infusion of CD34+/CD133 human umbilical-cord stem cells in Mexico (Fernando Ramirez, M.D.). We screened patient candidates for the study, made sure ethical standards and the highest standards of medical care were maintained, and then accrued and analyzed data concerning the responses of these eight children. At the end of the six-month study, it was found that all eight had experienced clinically and statistically significant improvements in at least seven areas of function. While not a rigorous clinical trial, this pilot study strongly suggests that such a trial is more than justified.

Among the more remarkable findings and observations we made: A four-year-old boy with cerebral palsy (CP) who was cortically blind and unable to speak or get about effectively prior to his treatment with 1.5 million umbilical-cord-derived stem cells, now does all three (www.prweb.com/releases/2005/2/prweb206140.htm). A six-year-old girl with CP and a smaller-than-average head (microcephaly) experienced impressive head growth and cognitive performance improvements in the year that followed her umbilical-cord stem-cell treatment. A recent quantitative electroencephalograph (qEEG) points to near normal function in areas of her brain that were dysfunctional prior to hUCSC therapy. Also, a seven-year-old girl with CP who was growth and developmentally delayed grew four inches and gained more than ten pounds in the first two months following hUCSC therapy, and went on to display motor skill improvements so striking as to prompt her physical therapist, Jill Conlon, P.T., M.H.S., to note, "My doubts about the effectiveness of stem-cell therapy are gone. Alyssa has demonstrated unbelievable growth in her abilities in just these three short months. *She is living proof* that this works [emphasis hers]. The changes in Alyssa's muscle tone have made it possible for her to perform volitional movements that she never did before. I realize it will take time to strengthen her muscles and help her to learn how to use them in more normal movement patterns, but now that her casts are off and I can work with her legs, the possibilities seem endless."

In addition and with special relevance to traumatic brain injury (TBI), our institute has been following four TBI patients (ages one to forty-two—mean age 19.5) who had a single infusion of umbilical-cord stem cells with three of the four showing moderate or better improvements in terms of motor performance, cognition, and balance (patient self-rating survey, 2005).

In assessing the suitability of stem cells for brain-injured soldiers, we note, first, what we at SRI and others have documented concerning favorable responses in brain-injured patients who have received human umbilical-cord stem cells. Second, there is cord blood's impressive track record in terms of safety—more than 5,000 cord-blood transplants medically employed for more than seventeen years for various cancer-related conditions that have consistently proven safe. (The world scientific literature indicates that even mismatched cord-blood infused into patients does not cause notable rejection—graft versus host disease.) Altogether, this record makes a clear and compelling logical imperative for pressing this type of stem cell into immediate use in treating America's soldiers, who have been brain injured on the battlefield. No harm will be done; there is at least a modicum of evidence now to suggest that human umbilical-cord blood-derived stem cells will bring about clinically significant improvements in our brain-injured soldiers, and the cost will be negligible. In other words, why wait for embryonic stem cells when this type of stem cell is available, safe, and in the hands of those who have used these cells clinically over the past few years—and these cells are more effective at reversing these types of brain injuries than anything else available?

Resources

Steenblock Research Institute
1064 Calle Negocio #B
San Clemente, CA 92673
Phone: 949-248-7034
Fax: 949-388-3441
Website: www.stemcelltherapies.org

David A. Steenblock, M.S., D.O.,
  President
E-mail: DrSteenblock@yahoo.com

Anthony G. Payne, Ph.D.,
  Resident Biological Theoretician
E-mail: biotheoretician@gmail.com

Brain Therapeutics Medical Clinic
26381 Crown Valley Parkway #130
Mission Viejo, CA 92691
Phone toll free: 800-300-1063 or
      949-367-8870
Website: www.strokedoctor.com

Fernando Ramirez, M.D.
Lloyd Building
Paseo Tijuana 406-Suite #203
Segunda Piso, Zona Del Rio
Tijuana, Baha California,
  Mexico C.P. 22310
Phone from the USA:
  011-5266-4973-2569
Website: www.ramirezdelrio.com
E-mail: RamirezDelRio@cox.net

PUBLIC CORD BLOOD BANKS

Celgene Corporation
86 Morris Avenue
Summit, NJ 07901
Phone: 908-673-9000
Website: www.celgene.com

Cryo-Banks International
270 S. Northlake Blvd., Suite 1012
Altamonte Springs, FL 32701
Phone: 407-834-8333 or
            800-869-8608
Fax: 407-834-3533
E-mail:
    clientservices@cryo-intl.com

National Marrow Donor
  Program
3001 Broadway Street Northeast,
  Suite 500
Minneapolis, MN 55413-1753

In the United States and Canada:
General information:
    800-MARROW2 (800-627-7692)
Office of Patient Advocacy (OPA):
    888-999-6743

Outside the United States and
  Canada:
General information:
    612-627-5800
Office of Patient Advocacy (OPA):
    612-627-8140
Website: www.marrow.org

PRIVATE CORD BLOOD BANKS

Alpha Cord, USA—Home Office
2200 Century Parkway #9
Atlanta, GA 30345
Phone: 866-396-7283
Fax: 404-795-9126
Website: www.alphacord.com

CellMed, Incorporated
1220 Commerce Street SW, Suite G
Conover, NC 28613
Phone: 828-466-2554 or
            866-460-2554
Fax: 828-466-2564
Website: www.cellmedbiotech.com

CorCell
1411 Walnut St., Suite 300
Philadelphia, PA 19102
Phone: 888-3-CORCELL
Website: www.corcell.com

Cord Blood Family Trust
400 Rolyn Place
Arcadia, CA 91007
Phone: 866-821-9820
    (office and storage in Arcadia, CA)
Website:
    www.cordbloodfamilytrust.com

Cord Blood Registry
1200 Bayhill Drive, Suite 301
San Bruno, CA 94066
Phone: 888-CORDBLOOD
    (office: San Bruno, CA;
    storage: Tucson, AZ)
Website: www.cordblood.com

CureSource
Affiliate of the Medical University of
South Carolina Foundation for
Research Development
65 Gadsden Street, Suite 200
Charleston, SC 29401-1192
Phone: 877-723-2247
Website: www.curesource.net/

Cryobanks International
270 S. Northlake Blvd., Suite 1012
Altamonte Springs, FL 32701
Phone: 407-834-8333 or
800-869-8608
Fax: 407-834-3533
E-mail: clientservices@cryo-intl.com
Website: www.cryo-intl.com

Cryo-Cell International
700 Brooker Creek Blvd.,
Suite 1800
Oldsmar, FL 34677
Phone: 1-800-STOR-CELL (office
and storage: Near Tampa, FL)
Website: www.cryo-cell.com

Family Cord Blood Services
3228 Nebraska Avenue
Santa Monica, CA 90404
Phone: 310-315-9402
(for Los Angeles residents)
or 800-400-3430
(outside Los Angeles and office
and storage, Santa Monica, CA)
Fax: 310-315-0472
Website: www.familycordblood
services.com

LifeLine Cryogenics
Health Sciences Building
1275 Summer Street, Suite 204
Stamford, CT 06905
Phone: 866-967-CRYO
(office and storage:
Stamford, CT)
Website:
www.lifelinecryogenics.com

MiraCell
1210 NE Windsor Drive
Lee's Summit, MO 64086
Phone: 816-554-5112
(office and storage: Lee's
Summit, MO)
Website: www.mira-cell.com

Newborn Blood Banking, Inc.
P.O. Box 270067
Tampa, Florida 33688
Phone: 888-948-CORD
(office and storage: Tampa, FL)
Website:
www.newbornblood.com

Viacord
245 First Street
Cambridge, MA 02142
Phone: 866-668-4895
(office: Boston, MA;
current storage: Hebron, KY,
outside Cincinnati)
Website: www.viacord.com

Selected References
and Notes

Umbilical-Cord Stem Cells:
Differentiation into Various Kinds of Cells

Baal, N., Reisinger, K., Jahr, H., et al., "Expression of transcription factor Oct-4 and other embryonic genes in CD133 positive cells from human umbilical cord blood," *Thromb Haemost* 92(4) (2004): 767–775.

Bicknese, A. R., Goodwin, H. S., Quinn, C.O., et al., "Human umbilical cord blood cells can be induced to express markers for neurons and glia," *Cell Transplant* 11(3) (2002): 261–264.

Buzanska, L., Machaj, E. K., Zablocka, et al., "Human cord blood-derived cells attain neuronal and glial features in vitro," *J Cell Sci* 115(Pt 10) (2002): 2131–2138.

Fu, Y. S., Shih, Y. T., Cheng, Y. C., et al., "Transformation of human umbilical mesenchymal cells into neurons in vitro," *J Biomed Sci* 11(5) (2004): 652–660.

Goodwin, H. S., Bichnese, A. R., Chien, S. N., et al., "Multilineage differentiation activity by cells isolated from umbilical cord blood: expression of bone, fat and neural markers," *Biol Blood Marrow Transplant* 7(11) (2001): 581–588.

Hao, S. G., Sun, G. L., Wu, W. L., et al., "Studies on the dynamics of biological characteristics of CD133+ cells from human umbilical cord blood during short-term culture," *Zhongguo Shi Yan Xue Ye Xue Za Zhi* 11(6) (2003): 569–575.

Hou, L., Cao, H., Wang, D., et al., "Induction of umbilical cord blood mesenchymal stem cells into neuron-like cells in vitro," *Int J Hematol* 778(3) (2003): 256–261.

Jang, Y. K., Par, J. J., Lee, M. C., et al., "Retinoic acid-mediated induction of neurons and glial cells from human umbilical cord-derived hematopoietic stem cells," *J Neurosci Res* 75(4) (2004): 573–584.

Jeong, J. A., Gang, E. J., Hong, S. H., et al., "Rapid neural differentiation of human cord blood-derived mesenchymal stem cells," *Neuroreport* 15(11) (2004): 1731–1734.

Kogler, G., Sensken, S., Airey, J. A., et al., "A new human somatic stem cell from placental cord blood with intrinsic pluripotent differentiation potential," *J Exp Med* 200(2) (2004): 223–235.

McGuckin, C. P., Forraz, N., Allouard, Q., et al., "Umbilical cord blood stem cells can expand hematopoietic and neuroglial progenitors in vitro," *Exp Cell Res* 295(2) (2004): 350–359.

Sanchez-Ramos, J. R., "Neural cells derived from adult bone marrow and umbilical cord blood," *J Neurosci Res* 69(6) (2002): 880–893.

Walczak, P., Chen, N., Hudson, J. E., et al., "Do hematopoietic cells exposed to a neurogenic environment mimic properties of endogenous neural precursors?" *J Neurosci Res* 76(2) (2004): 244–254.

Zhao, Z. M., Lu, S. H., Zhang, Q. J., et al., "The preliminary study on in vitro differentiation of human umbilical cord blood cells into neural cells," *Zhonghua Xue Ye Xue Za Zhi* 24(9) (2003): 484–487.

Zigova, T., Song, S., Willing, A. E., et al., "Human umbilical cord blood cells express neural antigens after transplantation into the developing rat brain," *Cell Transplant* 11(3) (2002): 265–274.

Heavy Metals Influence on Neurogenesis—A Sampling of Studies

Aaseth, J., Jacobsen, D., Andersen, O., et al., "Treatment of mercury and lead poisonings with dimercaptosuccinic acid (DMSA) and sodium dimercapto-propanesulfonate" (DMPS), *Analyst* 1995 Mar; 120: 853ff; presented at the Fifth Nordic Symposium on Trace Elements in Human Health and Disease, Loen, Norway, June 19–20, 1994.

Beers, M. H. and Berkow, M. D., *The Merck Manual of Diagnosis and Therapy.* Section 23 Chapter 307 Poisoning, Whitehouse Station, NJ: Merck & Co. 1999.

Chouchane, S. and Snow, E. T., "In vitro effect of arsenical compounds on glutathione-related enzymes," *Chem Res Toxicol* 14(5) (May 2001): 517–522.

Clarkson, T. W., "Mercury: An element of mystery," *N Engl J Med.* (1990): 1137–1139.

Daggett, E. A., Oberley, T. D., Nelson, S. A., et al., "Effects of lead on rat kidney and liver: GST-expression and oxidative stress," *Toxicology* 128(3) (17 July 1998): 191–206.

Dupler, D., "Heavy metal poisoning." *Gale Encyclopedia of Alternative Medicine.* Farmington Hills, MI: Gale Group 2001.

Faustman, E. M., Ponce, R. A., Ou, Y. C., et al., "Investigations of methyl mercury-induced alterations in neurogenesis," *Environ Health Perspect* 110 Suppl 5 (October 2002): 859–864.

Ferner, D. J., "Toxicity, heavy metals." *eMed J* 2(5) (25 May 2001): 1.

Gebel, T. and Dunkelberg, H., "Influence of chewing gum consumption and dental contact of amalgam fillings to different metal restorations on urine mercury content," *Zentralbl Hyg Umweltmed* 199(1) (November 1996): 69–75 (in German).

Goering, P. L., Aposhian, H. V., Mass, M. J., et al., "The enigma of arsenic carcinogenesis: role of metabolism," *Toxicol Sci* 49(1) (May 1999): 5–14.

Goyer, R. A., "Toxic effects of metals: mercury, in *"Casarett and Doull's Toxicology: The Basic Science of Poisons* 5th ed., New York: McGraw-Hill, 1996.

Ichimura, S., Report. General meeting of the Pharmaceutical Society of Japan, Hokuriku Branch, Toyoma City, Japan (27 October 1973).

International Occupational Safety and Health Information Centre. Chapter 7, "Metals," in *Basics of Chemical Safety.* Geneva: International Labour Organization, September 1999.

Isacsson, G., Barregard, L., Selden, A., et al., "Impact of nocturnal bruxism on mercury uptake from dental amalgams," *Eur J Oral Sci* 105(3) (June 1997): 251–257.

Klein-Schwartz, W. and Oderda, G. M., "Clinical toxicology," in *Textbook of Therapeutics: Drug and Disease Management,* 7th ed. Baltimore, MD: Williams & Wilkins, 2000, p. 51.

Maiti, S. and Chatterjee, A. K., "Effects on levels of glutathione and some related enzymes in tissues after an acute arsenic exposure in rats and their relationship to dietary protein deficiency," *Arch Toxicol* 75(9) (November 2001): 531–537.

Marcus, S., "Toxicity, lead," *eMed J* 2(6) (4 June 2001): 7.

Medical Management Guidelines (MMGs): *Managing Hazardous Material Incidents*, Volume III Atlanta, GA: Agency for Toxic Substances and Disease Registry, 2001 (http://www.atsdr.cdc.gov).

Mendoza, M. A., Ponce, R. A., Ou, Y. C., et al. "p21(WAF1/CIP1) inhibits cell cycle progression but not G2/M-phase transition following methyl mercury exposure," *Toxicol Appl Pharmacol* 178(2) (15 January 2002): 117–125.

Omura, Y., Shimotsuura, Y., Fukuoka, A., et al., "Significant mercury deposits in internal organs following the removal of dental amalgam, and development of pre-cancer on the gingiva and the sides of the tongue and their represented organs as a result of inadvertent exposure to strong curing light (used to solidify synthetic dental filling material) and effective treatment: a clinical case report, along with organ representation areas for each tooth," *Acupunct Electrother Res* 1(2) (1996): 133-160.

Roberts, J. R., "Metal toxicity in children," in *Training Manual on Pediatric Environmental Health: Putting It into Practice*. Emeryville, CA: Children's Environmental Health Network, June 1999 (www.cehn.org/cehn/trainingmanual/pdf/manual-full.pdf).

Sallsten, G., Thoren, J., Barregard, L., et al., "Long-term use of nicotine chewing gum and mercury exposure from dental amalgam fillings," *J Dent Res* 75(1) (January 1996): 594–598.

Saxe, S.R., Wekstein, M.W., Kryscio R., et al., "Alzheimer's disease, dental amalgam and mercury," *J Am Dent Assoc* 130(2) (February 1999): 191–199.

Segura Aguilar J., Kostrzewa, R. M., "Neurotoxins and neurotoxic species implicated in neurodegeneration," *Neurotox Res* 6(7–8) (2004): 615–630.

Shukla, G. S., Srivastava, R. S., and Chandra, S. V., "Glutathione status and cadmium neurotoxicity: studies in discrete brain regions of growing rats," *Fundam Appl Toxicol* 11(2) (August 1988): 229–235.

Sidhu, M., Sharma, M., Bhatia, M., et al., "Effect of chronic cadmium exposure on glutathione S-transferase and glutathione peroxidase activities in rhesus monkey: the role of selenium," *Toxicology* 83(1–3) (25 October 1993): 203–213.

Takeda, A., "Function and toxicity of trace metals in the central nervous system," *Clin Calcium* 14(8) (August 2004): 45–49.

ToxFAQs_for Aluminum. CAS 7429-90-5. Atlanta, GA: Agency for Toxic Substances and Disease Registry, June 1999.

ToxFAQs_for Arsenic. CAS 7440-38-2. Atlanta, GA: Agency for Toxic Substances and Disease Registry, July 2001.

ToxFAQs_for Cadmium. CAS 7440-43-9. Atlanta, GA: Agency for Toxic Substances and Disease Registry, June 1999.

ToxFAQs_for Lead. CAS 7439-92-1. Atlanta, GA: Agency for Toxic Substances and Disease Registry, June 1999.

ToxFAQs_for Mercury. CAS 7439-97-6. Atlanta, GA: Agency for Toxic Substances and Disease Registry, April 1999.

Tripathi, N. and Flora, S. J., "Effects of some thiol chelators on enzymatic activities in blood, liver and kidneys of acute arsenic (III) exposed mice," *Biomed Environ Sci* 11(1) (March 1998): 38–45.

Vij, A. G., Satija, N. K., and Flora, S.J., "Lead induced disorders in hematopoietic and drug metabolizing enzyme system and their protection by ascorbic acid supplementation," *Biomed Environ Sci* 11(1) (March 1998): 7–14.

Vimy, M. J., Takahashi, Y., Lorscheider, F. L., "Maternal-fetal distribution of mercury (203Hg) released from dental amalgam fillings," *Am J Physiol* 258(4, Pt. 2) (April 1990): R939–45.

Wentz, P. W., (LabCorp, Burlington, NC). "Chelation therapy: conventional treatments," in *Advance Magazines/Administrators of the Laboratory*. King of Prussia, PA: Merion, May 2000 (www.advanceforal.com/common/editorial/editorial/aspx).

West, W. L., Knight, E. M., Edwards, C. H., et al, "Maternal low level lead and pregnancy outcomes," *J Nutr* 124(6, Suppl.) (June 1994): 981S–986S.

WHO. "Aluminum," in *Guidelines for Drinking-Water Quality*, 2nd ed., Addendum to Volume 2, *Health Criteria and Other Supporting Information*. Geneva: World Health Organization, 1998, pp. 3–13.

Willershausen-Zonnchen, B., Zimmermann, M., Defregger, A., et al., "Mercury concentration in the mouth mucosa of patients with amalgam fillings," *Dtsch Med Wochenschr* 117(46) (13 November 1992): 1743–1747 (in German).

Wright, L. S., Kornguth, S. E., Oberley, T. D., et al., "Effects of lead on glutathione S-transferase expression in rat kidney: a dose-response study," *Toxicol Sci* 46(2) (December 1998): 254–259.

Yamanaka, K., Hayashi, H., Tachikawa, M., et al., "Metabolic methylation is a possible genotoxicity-enhancing process of inorganic arsenics," *Mutat Res* 394(1–3) (27 November 1997): 95–101.

Gut Dysbiosis-Bacterial, Fungal, Viral, and Other Causes and Contributors

Bartlett, J., "Antibiotic-associated diarrhea," *Clin Infect Dis* 15(1992):573–81.

Berg, R., "Promotion of enteric bacteria from the gastrointestinal tracts of mice by oral treatment with penicillin clindamycin, or metranidazole," *Infection and Immunity* 33(1981):854–861, 1981.

Finegold S. "Anaerobic infections and Clostridium difficile colitis emerging during antibacterial therapy," *Scand J Infect Dis* Suppl 49(1986): 160–164.

Fischer, A., Ballet, J., and Griscelli, C., "Specific inhibition of in vitro Candida-induced lymphocyte proliferation by polysaccharide antigens present in the serum of patients with chronic mucocutaneous candidiasis," *J Clin Invest* 62(1978): 1005–1013.

Gorbach, S., et al. "Successful treatment of relapsing Clostridium difficile colitis with Lactobacillus GG." *Lancet* (1987) ii: 1519.

Gupta, S., Aggarawal, S., and Heads, C., "Dysregulated immune system in children with autism. Beneficial effects of intravenous immune globulin on autistic characteristics," *J Autism Develop Dis* 26(1996): 439–452.

Hagerman, R. and Falkstein, A., "An association between recurrent otitis media in infancy and later hyperactivity." *Clin Pediat* 26(1987): 253–257.

Iwata, K. and Ichita, K., "Cellular immunity in experimental fungal infections in mice," *Mykosen Supplement* 1(1978): 72–81.

Kennedy, M. and Volz, P. "Dissemination of yeasts after gastrointestinal inoculation in antibiotic-treated mice." *Sabouradia* 21:27–33, 1983.

Kinsman O S, Pitblado K." Candida albicans gastrointestinal colonization and invasion in the mouse: effect of antibacterial dosing, antifungal therapy, and immunosuppression." *Mycoses* 32(1989):664–674.

Ostfeld, E., Rubinstein, E., Gazit, E., Smetana Z. "Effect of systemic antibiotics on the microbial flora of the external ear canal in hospitalized children." *Pediat* 60(1977): 364–366.

Roberts, J., Burchinal, M., and Campbell, F., "Otitis media in early childhood and patterns of intellectual development and later academic performance," *J Ped Psychol* 19(1994): 347–367.

Roboz, J. and Katz, R., "Diagnosis of disseminated candidiasis based on serum D/L arabinitol ratios using negative chemical ionization mass spectrometry," *J Chromatog* 575(1992): 281–286.

Sak, R. and Ruben, R., "Effects of recurrent middle ear effusion in preschool years on language and learning." *Developmental and Behavioral Pediatrics* 3 (1982): 7–11.

Samonis G., Gikas A., and Toloudis P., "Prospective evaluation of the impact of broad-spectrum antibiotics on the yeast flora of the human gut." *European Journal of Clinical Microbiology & Infectious Diseases* 13(1994):665–667.

Samonis, G.., Gikas, A., and Anaissie, E., "Prospective evaluation of the impact of broad-spectrum antibiotics on gastrointestinal yeast colonization of humans." *Antimicrobial Agents and Chemotherapy* 37(1993): 51–53.

Shah, D., and Larsen, B., "Identity of a Candida albicans toxin and its production in vaginal secretions," *Med Sci Res* 20(1992): 353–355.

Shaw W, Kassen E, and Chaves E. "Increased excretion of analogs of Krebs cycle metabolites and arabinose in two brothers with autistic features." *Clin Chem* 41(1995):1094–1104.

Shaw, W., Chaves, E., and Luxem, M., "Abnormal urine organic acids associated with fungal metabolism in urine samples of children with autism: preliminary results of a clinical trial with antifungal drugs." Published in The Proceedings of the Autism Society of American National Conference on Autism. Greensboro, NC, July 1995.

Shaw, W., "Organic acid testing: abnormal metabolites in the urine of children may assist in the diagnosis of, and therapies for, autism." Presented at the Autism Society of America National Conference on Autism, Las Vegas, NV, July 1994.

Shaw, W. and Chaves, E., "Experience with organic acid testing to evaluate abnormal microbial metabolites in the urine of children with autism." Published in *The Proceedings of the Autism Society of American National Conference on Autism*. Milwaukee, WI, 1996.

Silva, P., Chalmers, D., and Stewart, I., "Some audiological, psychological, educational, and behavioral characteristics of children with bilateral otitis media with effusion: a longitudinal study." *J Learning Disabilities* 19(1986): 165–169.

Singh, V. K., Frudenberg, H. H., Emerson, D., et al., "Immunodiagnosis and immunotherapy in autistic children," *Ann NY Acad Sci* 540(1998): 602–604.

Stubbs, E. G., Crawford, M. L., Burger, D. R., et al., "Depressed lymphocyte responsiveness in autistic children," *J Autism Child Schizophr* 7(1977): 49–55.

Sumiki Y. "Fermentation products of mold fungi. IV. *Aspergillus glaucus. I*," *J Agr Chem Soc Jap* 5(1929): 10.

Sumuki, Y., "Fermentation products of molds," *J Agr Chem Soc Jap* 7(1931): 819.

Teele, D., Klein, J., Rosner, B., and The Greater Boston Study Group. "Otitis media with effusion during the first years of life and development of speech and language." *Pediatrics* 74(1984): 282–287.

Van der Waaij, D., "Colonization resistance of the digestive tract—mechanism and clinical consequences." *Nahrung* 31(1987):507–517.

Varma, R. and Hoshino, A., "Serum glycoproteins in schizophrenia," *Carbohydrate Research* 82(1980): 343–351.

Varma, R., Michos, G.., Gordon, B., et al., "Serum glycoprotiens in children with schizophrenia and conduct and adjustment disorders," *Biochem Med* 30(1983): 206–214.

Vojdani, A., Rahimian, P., Kalhor, H., et al., "Immunological cross reactivity between candida albicans and human tissue." *J Clin Lab Immunol* 48(1996): 1–15.

Warren, R. P., Foster, A., Margaretten, N. C., "Immune abnormalities in patients with autism," *J Autism Develop Dis* 16(1986): 189–197.

Warren, R. P., Yonk, J., Burger, R. A., et al., "Dr. positive T cells in autism: association with decreased plasma levels of the complement C4B protein," *Neurophyschobiology* 39(1995): 53–57.

Dietary Influences on Stem Cells, Neurogenesis, etc.

Chu, Y. F., Sun, J., Wu, X., et al., "Antioxidant and antiproliferative activities of common vegetables," *J Agric Food Chem.* 50(23) (6 November 2002): 6910–6916.

Sun, J., Chu, Y.F., Wu, X., et al., "Antioxidant and antiproliferative activities of common fruits," *J Agric Food Chem.* 50(25) (4 December 2002): 7449–7454.

Grains and Inflammation

Kanauchi, O., Serizawa, I., Araki, Y., et al., "A type 1 diabetes-related protein from wheat (Triticum aestivum): cDNA clone of a wheat storage globulin, Glb1, linked to islet damage," *J Biol Chem* 278(1) (3 January 2003): 54–63. Epub. October 29, 2002.

Otsuka, M., Yamaguchi, K., and Ueki, A., "Similarities and differences between Alzheimer's disease and vascular dementia from the viewpoint of nutrition," *Ann N Y Acad Sci* 977 (November 2002): 155–161.

Takaki, K., Toyonaga, A., Sata, M., et al., "Germinated barley foodstuff, a prebiotic product, ameliorates inflammation of colitis through modulation of the enteric environment," *J Gastroenterol* 38(2) (2003): 134–141.

Turturro, A., Duffy, P., Hass, B., et al., "Survival characteristics and age-adjusted disease incidences in C57BL/6 mice fed a commonly used cereal-based diet modulated by dietary restriction," *J Gerontol A Biol Sci Med Sci* 57(11) (November 2002): B379–389.

Grains and Opioids and Stem Cells

Bell, I. R., Schwartz, G. E., Peterson, J. M., et al., "Symptom and personality profiles of young adults from a college student population with self-reported illness from foods and chemicals," *J Am Coll Nutr* 12(6) (1993): 693–702.

The present study investigated self-reported illness from several common foods—wheat, dairy and eggs—and indigestion, headache, and memory problems. The illness groups reported significantly more limitation of foods that mobilize endogenous opioids or generate exogenous opioids (sweets, fats, bread) as well as more illness from opiate drugs, small amounts of beverage alcohol, and late meals.

Hauser, K. F., Houdi, A. A., Turbek, C. S., et al., "Opioids intrinsically inhibit the genesis of mouse cerebellar granule neuron precursors in vitro: differential impact of mu and delta receptor activation on proliferation and neurite elongation," *Eur J Neurosci.* 12(4) (April 2000): 1281–1293.

Horowitz, D., Callahan, J.F., Pelus, L.M., et al., "Inhibition of hematopoietic progenitor cell growth by Tyr-MIF, an endogenous opiate modulator, and its degradation products," *Int Immunopharmacol* 2(5) (April 2002): 721–730.

There is increasing evidence that neuronal factors can affect hematopoietic cell proliferation. Endogenous opioids with specificity for several opioid receptor classes were tested for their ability to inhibit murine and human hematopoietic progenitor cell proliferation. Tyr-MIF, an opioid tetrapeptide (H-Tyr-Pro-Leu-Gly-NH2), demonstrated a dose-dependent inhibition of colony formation at concentration.

Knapp, P. E., Itkis, O. S., Zhang, L., et al., "Endogenous opioids and oligodendroglial function: possible autocrine/paracrine effects on cell survival and development," *Glia* 35(2) (August 2001): 156–165.

Persson, A. I., Thorlin, T., Bull, C., et al., "Mu- and delta-opioid receptor antagonists decrease proliferation and increase neurogenesis in cultures of rat adult hippocampal progenitors," *Eur J Neurosci* 17(6) (March 2003): 1159–1172.

Roy, S., Loh and H.H., "Effects of opioids on the immune system," *Neurochem Res.* 21(11) (November 1996): 1375–1386.

Schick, R. and Schusdziarra, V., "Physiological, pathophysiological and pharmacological aspects of exogenous and endogenous opiates," *Clin Physiol Biochem*, 3(1) (1985): 43–60.

Opioid active peptides have been found in certain nutrients such as wheat gluten and bovine and human milk.

Whole Grains and Reduced Insulin

Braly, J. and Hoggan, R., *Dangerous Grains*. New York, NY: Avery Books, 2002.

Koh-Banerjee, P. and Rimm, E.B., "Whole grain consumption and weight gain: a review of the epidemiological evidence, potential mechanisms and opportunities for future research," *Proc Nutr Soc.* 62(1) (February 2003): 25–29.

Animal Model: Alzheimer's Disease

Ende, N., Chen, R., and Ende-Harris, D., "Human umbilical cord blood cells ameliorate Alzheimer's disease in transgenic mice," *J Med*, 32(3–4) (2001): 241–247.

Having had success in extending the life of mice with a transgene for amyotropic lateral sclerosis mice and Huntington's disease, we administered megadoses of human umbilical-cord blood mononuclear cells to mice with Alzheimer's disease. These mice have an over-expression of human Alzheimer amyloid precursor protein, die early and develop a CNS disorder that included neophobia. When given 110 x 10 (6) human umbilical-cord blood mononuclear cells, these mice had considerable extension of life with a p value of 0.001 when compared to control animals.

Animal Model: Amyotrophic Lateral Sclerosis

Garbuzova-Davis, S., Willing, A. E., Zigova, T., et al., "Intravenous administration of human umbilical cord blood cells in a mouse model of amyotrophic lateral sclerosis: distribution, migration and differentiation." *J Hematother Stem Cell Res* 12(3) (2003): 255–270.

The authors studied the long-term effects of the intravenous administration of umbilical-cord blood cells in a mouse model of amyotrophic lateral sclerosis. The treat-

ment in presymptomatic G93A mice resulted in a delay of the disease progression by two to three weeks and an increased lifespan in the diseased mice. In addition, the transplanted cells survived ten to twelve weeks after administration and entered regions of motor neuron degeneration in the brain and spinal cord. There, the cells expressed neural markers (nestin, III Beta-Tubulin, and glial fibrilary acidic protein). The transplanted cells were also widely distributed in the peripheral circulation and organs, mainly the spleen.

Animal Model: Huntington's Disease

Ende, N. and Chen, R., "Human umbilical cord blood cells ameliorate Huntington's disease in transgenic mice," *J Med* 32(3–4) (2001): 231–240.

Human umbilical-cord blood mononuclear cells given in megadose quantity were able to increase the life span of B₆CBA-TgN 62 Gpb mice (Huntington's disease) from an average of 88 days to 97.8 and 103.4 days respectively. The rate of weight loss, which begins in these mice before the onset of symptoms of chorea, was far less in the animals receiving human cord-blood mononuclear cells than the weight loss in untreated control mice.

Animal Model: Stroke

Cairns, K. and Finklestein, S. P., "Growth factors and stem cells as treatments for stroke recovery," *Phys Med Rehabil Clin N Am* 14(1 Suppl) (2003): S135–142.

Growth factors and stem-cell populations from bone-marrow and umbilical-cord blood hold promise as treatments to enhance neurological recovery after stroke. Growth factors may exert their effects through stimulation of neural sprouting and enhancement of endogenous progenitor cell proliferation, migration, and differentiation in the brain. Treatments with stem cells may act as miniature "factories" for growth factors in the poststroke brain. Recovery in chronic stroke represents an important and under-explored opportunity for the development of new stroke treatments.

Chen, J., Sanberg, P., Li, Y., et al., "Intravenous administration of human umbilical cord blood reduces behavioral deficits after stroke in rats," *Stroke*, 32 (2001): 2682–2688.

Human umbilical-cord blood cells (hUCBC) are rich in stem and progenitor cells. In this study the authors tested whether intravenously infused cord-blood cells can enter the brain, survive, differentiate, and improve neurological functional recovery after stroke is induced in rats. Twenty-four hours after treating stroke-induced rats with hUCBC, the rats were showing functional recovery. Significant hUCBC migration activity was present at twenty-four hours after stroke compared with the normal brain tissue (in vitro). This study was one of the first to demonstrate that intra-venously administered human umbilical-cord blood cells are able to enter the brain, survive, migrate, and improve functional recovery after stroke.

Peterson, D. A., "Umbilical cord blood cells and brain stroke injury: bringing in fresh blood to address an old problem," *J Clin Invest* 114(3) (2004): 312–324.

Evidence suggests that the delivery of human umbilical-cord stem cells (CD34+) can produce functional recovery in an animal stroke model by the cells assisting with the development of both new blood vessels and new neurons in the brain, thereby leading to some degree of brain repair.

Taguchi, A., Soma, T., Tanaka, H., et al. "Administration of CD34+ cells after stroke enhances neurogenesis via angiogenesis in a mouse model," *J Clin Invest* 114(3) (2004): 330–338.

Immunocompromised mice were subjected to stroke and then given human cord blood-derived (CD34+) cells. Forty-eight hours later there was already new blood-vessel development in the brain tissue that had been damaged, new neural growth was under way, and neural stem/progenitor cells had migrated to the damaged area. The authors suggested that CD34+ cells create a microenvironment that is conducive to new blood-vessel growth in damaged brain tissue such that neuronal regeneration can proceed.

Willing, A. E., Lixian, J., Milliken, M., Poulos, S., et al., "Intravenous versus intrastriatal cord-blood administration in a rodent model of stroke," *J Neurosci Res* 73(3) (2003): 296–307.

Human umbilical-cord stem cells were administered intravenously into the femoral (leg) vein or directly into the brain (striatum) of rats with induced strokes. It was found that behavioral recovery was similar with both methods of delivery. However, with the step test, greater improvement was seen with the femoral delivery. The results suggest that therapy with umbilical-cord stem cells may be effective for brain injuries and neurodegenerative disorders, and that intravenous administration may be more effective than striatal implantation for long-term functional improvement in stroke animal models.

Animal Model: Traumatic Brain Injury

Lu, D., Sanberg, P. R., Mahmood, A., et al., "Intravenous administration of human umbilical cord blood reduces neurological deficit in the rat after trau-matic brain injury," *Cell Transplant* 11(3) (2002): 275–281.

Human umbilical-cord blood was administered intravenously in the tail vein of rats twenty-four hours after TBI. The cord blood cells significantly reduced motor and neurological deficits compared with control animals by the 28th day. The cells preferentially entered the brain, migrated into the injured area and expressed markers for neurons (NeuN and MAP-2) and markers for astrocytes (GFAP). Some cord-blood cells also integrated into the vascular walls within the injured area. The results suggest that human umbilical-cord blood may be useful for treating TBI.

Newman, M. B., Davis, C. D., Kuzmin-Nichols, N., et al., "Human umbilical cord blood (HUCB) cells for central nervous system repair," *Neurotox Res* 5(5) (2003): 355–368.

The hematopoietic system offers alternative sources for stem cells compared to those of fetal or embryonic origin. Umbilical-cord cells and bone-marrow stromal cells have been used in preclinical models of brain injury; they have been directed to differentiate into neural phenotypes, and they have been related to functional recovery after engraftment in central nervous system injury models.

Sanberg, P. R., Willing, A. E., and Cahill, D. W., "Novel cellular approaches to repair of neurodegenerative disease: from Sertoli cells to umbilical cord blood stem cells," *Neurotox Res* 4(2) (2002): 95–101.

The authors review the possible alternative cell sources for repair of the brain and spinal cord, including Sertoli cells, neurotrophics, bone marrow, and umbilical-cord blood-derived stem cells.

Notes

Chapter 7: Natural Methods of Stem-Cell Renewal

1. Altman, J. and Das, G. D., "Post-natal origin of microneurones in the rat brain," *Nature* 207 (1965): 953–956.

2. Green, P., Rohling, M. L., Iverson G. L., et al., "Relationships between olfactory discrimination and head injury severity," *Brain Injury* 17(6) (2003): 479–496.

3. Tabert, M. H., Liu, X., Doty, R. L., et al., "A 10-item smell identification scale related to risk for Alzheimer's disease," *Annals of Neurology* 58(1) (2005): 155–160.

4. Sapolsky, R. M., "Glucocorticoids, stress and their adverse neurological effects: Relevance to aging," *Experimental Gerontology*, 34 (1999): 721–732.

5. Oben, J. A., Roskams, T., Yang, S., et al., "Sympathetic nervous system inhibition increases hepatic progenitors and reduces liver injury," *Hepatology* 38(3) (2003): 664–73.

6. Aleksandrin, V. V., Tarasova, N. N., and Tarakanov I. A., "Effect of serotonin on respiration, cerebral circulation and blood pressure in rat,." *Bulletin of Experimental Biology and Medicine* 139(1) (2005): 64–67.

7. Palmer, T. D., Colamarino, S., Gage, F. H., "Mobilizing endogenous stem cells," in Rao, M. (ed.) *Stem Cells and CNS Development*, Totowa, NJ: Humana Press, 2001, pp. 263–289.

8. Banasr, M., Hery, M., Brezun, J. M., et al., "Serotonin mediates oestrogen stimulation of cell proliferation in the adult dentate gyrus," *European Journal of Neuroscience* 14 (2001): 1417–1424.

9. Kim, M. J., Kim, H. K., Kim, B.S., et al., "Melatonin increases cell proliferation in the dentate gyrus of maternally separated rats," *Journal of Pineal Research* 37(3) (2004): 193–197.

10. Tung, A., Takase, L., Fornal, C., et al., "Effects of Sleep Deprivation and Recovery Sleep upon Cell Proliferation in Adult Rat Dentate Gyrus," *Neuroscience* 134(3) (2005): 721–723.

11. Karasek, M., "Melatonin, human aging, and age-related diseases," *Experimental Gerontology* 39 (2004): 1723–1729.

12. Reiter, R. J, Tan, D.-X., and Pappolla, M. A., "Melatonin relieves the neural oxidative burden that contributes to dementia," *Annals of the New York Academy of Sciences* 1035 (2004): 179–196.

13. Colao, A., Di Somma, C., Cuocolo ,A., et al., "The severity of growth hormone deficiency correlates with the severity of cardiac impairment in 100 adult patients with hypopituitarism: an observation, case-control study," *J Clinical Endocrinology and Metabolism* 89(12) (2004): 5998–6004.

14. Ariznavarreta, C., Castillo, C., Segovia, G., et al. "Growth hormone and aging," *Hormones* 53(2) (2003): 132–141.

15. Urban, R. J., Harris, P, Masel, B., "Anterior hypopituitarism following traumatic brain injury," *Brain Injury* 19(5) (2005): 349–358.

16. Matarredona, E. R., Murillo-Carretero, M., Moreno-López, B., et al., "Nitric oxide synthesis inhibition increases proliferation of neural precursors isolated from the postnatal mouse subventricular zone," *Brain Research* 995 (2004): 274–284.

17. Buzzard, A. R., Peng, Q., Lau, B. H., "Kyolic® and pycnogenol® increase human growth hormone secretion in genetically-engineered keratinocytes." *Growth Hormone and IGF Research* 12(1) (2002, February): 34–40.

18. Barbagallo S. G., Barbagallo M., Giordano M., et al., "Alpha-glycerophospho-choline in the mental recovery of cerebral ischemic attacks: an Italian multicenter clinical trial," Annals *of the New York Academy of Sciences* 717 (1994): 253–269.

19. Coiro, V., Volpi, R., Capretti, L., et al., "Inhibition of growth hormone secretion in mild primary hyperparathyroidism," *Hormone Research* 62(2) (2004): 88–91.

20. Féron, F., Burne, T. H. J., Brown, J., et al., "Developmental vitamin D$_3$ deficiency alters the adult rat brain," *Brain Research Bulletin* 65 (2005): 141–148.

21. Nakagawa, T., Tsuchida, A., Itakura, Y., et al., "Brain-derived neurotrophic factor regulates glucose metabolism by modulating energy balance in diabetic mice," *Diabetes* 49(3) (2000): 436–444.

22. Wirz-Justice, A., Benedetti, F., Berger, M., et al., "Chronotherapeutics (light and wake therapy) in affective disorders," *Psychol Med* 35(7) (2005): 939–944.

23. Turek, F. W., "Role of light in circadian entrainment and treating sleep disorders—and more," *Sleep* 28(5) (2005): 548–549.

24. Wang, Y., Chiang, Y.-H., Su,T.-P., et al., "Vitamin D$_3$ attenuates cortical infarction induced by middle cerebral arterial ligation in rats," *Neuropharmacology* 39 (2000): 873–880.

25. Wang, J.-Y., Wu, J.-N, Cherng,.T.-L., et al., "Vitamin D$_3$ attenuates 6-hydroxydopamine-induced neurotoxicity in rats," *Brain Research* 904 (2001): 67–75.

26. Bruel-Jungerman, E., Laroche, S., and Rampon, C., "New neurons in the dentate gyrus are involved in the expression of enhanced long-term memory following environmental enrichment," *European Journal of Neuroscience* 21 (2005): 513-521.

27. Schmidt-Hieber, C., Jonas, P., and Bischofberger, J. "Enhanced synaptic plasticity in newly generated granule cells of the adult hippocampus," *Nature* 429 (2004): 184–187.

28. Lazarov, O., Robinson, J., Tang Y.-P., et al., "Environmental enrichment

reduces AB levels and amyloid deposition in transgenic mice," *Cell* 120 (2005): 701–713.

29. Komitova, M., Zhao, L. R., Gido, G., et al., "Postischemic exercise attenuates whereas enriched environment has certain enhancing effects on lesion-induced subventricular zone activation in the adult rat," *European Journal of Neuroscience* 21 (2005): 2397–2405.

30. Karten, Y. J. G., Olariu, A., and Cameron H. A., "Stress in early life inhibits neurogenesis in adulthood," *Trends in Neurosciences* 28(4) (2005): 171–172.

31. Coe, C. L., Kramer, M., Czeh, B., et al., "Prenatal stress diminishes neurogenesis in the dentate gyrus of juvenile rhesus monkeys," *Biological Psychiatry* 54(10) (2003): 1025–1034.

32. Fiore, M., Amendola, T., Triaca, V., et al., "Agonistic encounters in aged male mouse potentiate the expression of endogenous brain NGF and BDNF: Possible implication for brain progenitor cells' activation," *European Journal of Neuroscience* 17 (2003): 1455–1464.

33. Cotman, W. and Berchtold, N. C., "Exercise: A behavioral intervention to enhance brain health and plasticity," *Trends in Neurosciences* 25(6) (2002): 295–301.

34. Lee, J., Duan, W., and Mattson, M. P. "Evidence that brain-derived neurotrophic factor is required for basal neurogenesis and mediates, in part, the enhancement of neurogenesis by dietary restriction in the hippocampus of adult mice," *Journal of Neurochemistry* 82 (2002): 1367–1375.

35. Matou, S., Helley, D., Chabut, D., et al., "Effect of fucoidan on fibroblast growth factor-2-induced angiogenesis in vitro," *Thrombosis Research* 106 (2002): 213–221.

36. Frenette, P. S. and Weiss, L. "Sulfated glycans induce rapid hematopoietic progenitor cell mobilization: evidence for selectin-dependent and independent mechanisms. *Blood* 96 (2000): 2460–2468.

37. Edelberg, J. M., Tang, L., Hattori, K., et al., "Young adult bone marrow-derived endothelial precursor cells restore aging-impaired cardiac angiogenic function," *Circulation Reseach* 90 (2002): e89–e93.

38. Six, I., Gasan, G., Mura, E., et al., "Beneficial effect of pharmacological mobilization of bone marrow in experimental cerebral ischemia," *European Journal of Pharmacology* 458 (2003): 327–328.

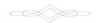

Index

About Steenblock
Research Institute (SRI)

- Founded in 2003 with a staff of two; now with a staff of seven, including a statistician, chemist, lab tech, and medical librarian.

- 501(c) 3 nonprofit status granted during 2004.

- 12,000-plus volume medical and scientific library.

- In-house laboratory doing ELISA and other laboratory tests.

- Developed USPTO Patent Pending protocols for pre- and post-hUCSC therapy.

- Accrued data and case history documentation on more than 125 patients treated with hUCSCs in Mexico.

- In October 2004, asked by the White House (William Chatfield, Director of Selective Service http://www.sss.gov/ChatfieldBIO.htm) to provide input on human umbilical cord stem cells to President George Bush.

- Provides technical support and data analysis to research-oriented clinic-based hUCSC therapy programs in Mexico, including a pilot study headed up by Fernando Ramirez, M.D., in which eight children with cerebral were treated with hUCSCs in 2004. All eight experienced clinically significant improvements in seven areas of function, with resolution of cortical blindness in a four-year-old boy, Adam Susser, three months after his treatment. This is discussed in a paper published in *Medical Hypotheses & Research Journal*:

A.G. Payne [2005] *Med Hypotheses Res* 2:497-501, "Beneficial Effects of Subcutaneously Injected Human Umbilical Cord Stem Cells on Cerebral Palsy and Traumatic Brain Injury in Children and a Posited Mechanism" www.journal-mhr.com/PDF_Files/vol_2_3/ 2_3_PDFs/2_3_6.pdf

- Helped launch the creation of ARS-A gene transvected hUCSCs to treat the terminal neurologic condition metachromatic leukodystrophy, as well as interleukin-2 and gamma-interferon gene transvected hUCSCs specific for treating cancer.

About the Authors

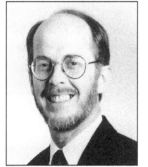

David A. Steenblock, M.S., D.O., is the Founder and Director of the Brain Therapeutics Medical Clinic in Mission Viejo, California, which began in 1978, and President of Steenblock Research Institute, a 501(c) (3) nonprofit organization devoted to education and research in the cause of advancing the human condition.

He began his scientific career in the Department of Zoology at Iowa State University where he was the recipient of a National Science Foundation Undergraduate Research Participant Award for his work on neuromuscular synaptic physiology from 1963 to 1969.

In graduate school (1964–1967), he completed his Masters of Science (MS) degree in Biochemistry on the regulation of the blood-clotting system and its role in the development of atherosclerosis.

Throughout medical school, Dr. Steenblock directed the research activities of the biochemistry laboratory at the College of Osteopathic Medicine in Des Moines, Iowa. His post-doctoral training included three years at Case Western Reserve University, one year at the Oregon Health Sciences University, and a clinical Rotating Internship at Providence Hospital in Seattle, Washington.

In April 2002, Dr. Steenblock was awarded the Charles M. Farr Award by the International Oxidative Medicine Association for his pioneering work in oxidative medicine.

Dr. Steenblock has devoted many years to research in the fields of biochemistry, pathology, nerve and muscle physiology, cardiovascular disease and other diseases of aging. He has also written numerous scientific articles and is a contributing editor to several national consumer health magazines.

Dr. Steenblock's Curriculum Vitae (c.v.) can be found at www.strokedoctor.com and some of his papers on hUCSCs on www.stem cclltherapies.org.

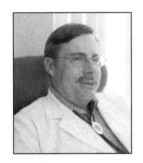

Anthony G. Payne, Ph.D., is a biological theoretician and senior science writer on staff at Steenblock Research Institute. He holds undergraduate and graduate degrees in biological anthropology, plus doctorates in both nutritional medicine (emphasizing Darwinian nutrition) and theocentric psychology (with a focus on Cognitive Therapy, and Darwinian or evolutionary psychology). A native Texan (hometown: Plainview), Dr. Payne is a U.S. Bureau of Indian Affairs certified American Indian, a member of the Choctaw Tribe (Nation) of Oklahoma (www.choctawnation.com), and a twenty-plus-year member of the international high IQ/genius society, MENSA. Prior to joining the staff of SRI, Dr. Payne spent many years working as a bench-top researcher, scientific consultant, and technical writer for numerous U.S. companies; he then spent four years teaching at various schools in Japan including Teikyo University of Science & Technology, Asia University, and Toshiba Institute. He and his Japanese wife, Sachi, live in southern California. Many of Dr. Payne's papers, essays, and other works can be found on http://14ushop.com/wizard.